THE
SMILING
DENTIST

What People Are Saying

"I have owned Oakdale dental for eight years and did not want just anybody to take over. When I first met Alif I knew he would be the right person. He has great knowledge and ability as a dentist but more importantly he is kind, caring and patient. These are the qualities you need to have a great chair side manner and to really help patients. If you can not listen and communicate effectively as a dentist, you will never know what your patient wants and so you will never be able to deliver. At Oakdale dental we strive to put the patient first and always make sure we deliver. That is why Alif was the natural choice to succeed me as Clinical Director at such a prestigious practice but also the right person to write this book."

—Mr. Bayan Al Sarraj BDS. FDS,RCPS (Glasg), Specialist in Oral Surgery | ITI mentor

"Alif is a great dentist but he is also a fantastic teacher. I remember when we studied together as dental students. He was always the one that people used to go to to help explain difficult concepts in a simple, understandable and accessible way. He is definitely the right person to have written this book. The book that makes the knowledge that dentist's have accessible to all."

—Dr. Hanel Nathwani BDS, Harley Street Dentist as featured on Channel 4's '10 Years Younger' | star of Sensodyne adverts

"I met Alif on many occasions at Post-Graduate courses and find him a hugely committed young dentist who is pursuing a course of excellence to try and make himself the best practitioner possible.

"I was given an advance copy of his book 'The Smiling Dentist' and was fascinated by the concept of writing a book for patient information, which would be ideal for waiting rooms and to give patients ideas on informed treatment choices. I think this is a great idea, it's not a "big sell" and is a very useful tool for patients to make informed decisions regarding their treatment which I think is the only way forward for our profession.

"The book also donates it's profits to Bridge2Aid which I am a huge supporter of so I wish Alif the best of luck with this excellent project and would advise anyone to pay attention to this when they come across it."

—Colin Campbell BDS FDSRCS Specialist in Oral Surgery | ITI Fellow

"Looking after your teeth is so simple, but so important. The consequences of not doing so are painful and debilitating. Thankfully in the UK there is a great book like 'The Smiling Dentist' to advise us, and skilful dentists like Alif to turn to.

"The communities we work within East Africa have no-one to help them, which is why our work training local health workers to provide simple treatment is life changing. More of it will be made possible by the generous contribution from Alif, and we're extremely grateful for his support."

—Mark Topley, CEO Bridge2Aid

I dedicate this book to my parents, to my wife, and to my daughter.

To my wonderful, happy and supportive parents, Bakirali and Rashida, who put me on the path to success when I was very young.
You have instilled the work ethic that I carry with me today. Without that, none of this would have been possible.

To my beautiful, loving and supportive wife, Rumana, who taught me never to accept a lesser version of myself, to always aim higher than you think you should, and to always dream big, stop, then dream bigger!
Without your lessons, none of this would have been possible.

To my adorable, sweet darling daughter, Anniyah (Anni) who loves me unconditionally and who had my heart the moment I saw her. You gave me the reason I needed to succeed without even the notion of failing. I hope you will be proud of me.
Without your love and that motivation, none of this would have been possible.

Foreword by Raymond Aaron

- Are you afraid of going to the dentist?
- Do you always have to have fillings when you go to the dentist and don't know why?
- Do your gums bleed?
- Does your breath smell?
- Are you worried about your children's teeth?
- Would you like to know what to do if your child knocked a tooth out?
- Are you a nervous dental patient?

Well, if you have answered "yes" to any of the above questions, then this is the book for you.

It will answer all of these questions and many more in a very clear and thorough way.

This book will also explain exactly what dentists do and the reason why they carry out the treatment that they do.

If you are fearful of going to the dentist because you don't know what's going on in your mouth, then after you've read this book, you can say goodbye to that uncertainty.

Dr Alif Moosajee, the Smiling Dentist, is also the dentist with a difference.

He genuinely cares not only about the quality of his treatment but also about the quality of the experience that his patients have.

He feels that by communicating effectively with you, he can impart the knowledge that can put you at ease. That is why Dr. Moosajee is able to write this book so well. This brilliant, clear, concise, and jargon-free book finally gives you the secrets of having great teeth.

Yours faithfully
Raymond Aaron
New York Times best-selling author

Introduction

When I set out to write this book, I wanted to answer the questions that patients really ask me most frequently. That is why the chapter titles are the genuine questions I get asked by patients that sit in my chair every day.

I thought, if these are the questions that my patients frequently wanted answered, then I could write a book providing the answers that I frequently give. Perhaps the people who do not come and see me or those who are too afraid to ask, may also have access to the knowledge that I share with my patients on a daily basis.

I do hope you will read all of the book (and enjoy it) however, I have set up the book so that if there is a specific question that you have, you can look it up in the table of contents and read the chapter pertaining to that question.

If I have not covered a topic you have a question about in this book, please contact me. You can email me by visiting my website www.smilingdentist.co.uk or you can contact me on my Facebook page www.facebook.com/smilingdentist.

I look forward to hearing from you and hope to maybe even see you or treat you one day.

Yours faithfully
Dr. Alif Moosajee BDS (Birm) MFGDP(UK) MJDF(RCS Eng)
The Smiling Dentist

bridge2aid

75% of the world's population has no access to a Dentist. Dental charity Bridge2Aid is working to change this by providing emergency dental training for Health Workers in developing nations. So far, Bridge2Aid has trained over 300 workers in East Africa, creating safe and sustainable access to treatment for over 3 million people in rural communities.

All of the profits from this book will be donated to Bridge2Aid.

www.bridge2aid.org

THE
SMILING
DENTIST

Secrets from a top dentist on how to keep your
smile looking younger and healthier for longer

DR. ALIF MOOSAJEE

Table of Contents

Chapter 1

"My Gums Bleed, What Should I Do?"

The 5 most common mistakes when cleaning your teeth and how to avoid them.

Mistake 1: Trauma Does Not Cause Gums to Bleed: Bacteria Does

The human mouth is full of bacteria and these bacteria aggregate or clump together to form a biofilm that we call 'plaque'. Plaque is that soft, white stuff you can scrape off your teeth when you wake up in the morning. Removing it is the reason we brush our teeth.

Essentially, plaque is like a soft wall where the bacteria are the bricks and the toxic products they produce are the cement. These bacteria produce toxins which are very harmful to the gums, and more importantly the bone that normally holds the teeth firmly.

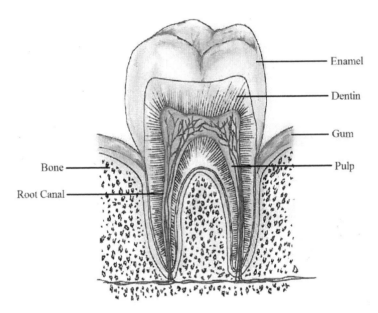

Enamel

Dentin

Gum

Bone

Pulp

Root Canal

ILLUSTRATION OF THE ANATOMY OF A TOOTH: THE RELATIONSHIP BETWEEN THE TOOTH, THE GUM AND THE BONE CAN BE SEEN.

The toxins cause a process called 'inflammation' which is really another word for irritation. Inflammation causes the gums to look red and swollen and to bleed. The gums bleed because inflammation results in an increased blood supply to the area that is irritated. The blood carries cells which normally help to fight the infection and help repair the affected area. Unfortunately, in the gums this does not really cure the problem, and all that is left are gums which bleed more readily than they should.

Often, people will avoid brushing areas that bleed in the hope that the bleeding will stop. This only serves to make matters worse, though, because this means that even more plaque stagnates, and the bleeding and the rest of the disease process only gets worse

The toxins can also cause the bone to shrink away or 'resorb'. If this loss of bone is allowed to continue, the tooth will no longer have the foundation or the support that it needs and eventually it will start to wobble up. This is the process that happens in 'periodontal disease' or 'Periodontitis'. It is the most common cause of tooth loss and is the reason why dentists tell people to brush twice a day and why we insist on cleaning the teeth every time you come to visit us for an examination.

I mentioned how the bacteria form a wall because I have had patients ask me if it is enough to just rinse the mouth with mouthwash without brushing. I explain that the mouthwash cannot penetrate that wall and it must be broken up mechanically; and that is where effective tooth brushing and inter-dental (between the teeth) cleaning is important. Mouthwash can be useful in removing the free-floating bacteria that can remain after brushing, but it is an aid to a process and not to be thought of as the only step.

Mistake 2: Wrong Angulation of the Brush

I see many very good patients who are regular attenders, and care about the health of their teeth and gums. They also tell me that they brush at least twice a day, every day. However, when I look in their mouths there is still a lot of plaque visible and the gums do bleed and are definitely inflamed. When I see this, I am sure that there is a problem with the technique they use for brushing, so I instruct them on this to improve it.

Plaque accumulates mostly around the margin where the gum meets the tooth.

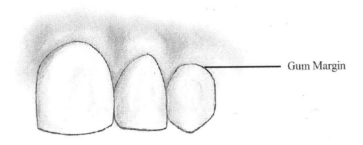

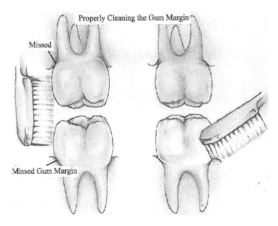

ILLUSTRATION THE POSITION OF THE GUM MARGIN RELATIVE TO THE TOOTH AND GUM

There is a technique for brushing called the 'Modified Bass Technique' which is the gold standard for brushing. I like to break this technique down into three small tips which I will discuss now.

If the toothbrush is held flat against the tooth, it is very easy to miss the 'Gingival margin'. This is the bit where the gum meets the tooth, the bit that is really important. So **Tip number 1** is to angle or rotate the brush up 45 degrees for the top teeth and down 45 degrees for the lower teeth. This means that the bristles of the brush are removing the plaque from the most important area (i.e. the gum margin).

ILLUSTRATION SHOWING INCORRECT BRUSHING TECHNIQUE ON THE LEFT AND HOW EASY IT IS TO MISS THE GUM MARGIN OF THE TOOTH WHEN BRUSHING WITH THE TOOTH BRUSH FLAT AGAINST THE TEETH. ON THE RIGHT SHOWING CORRECT ANGULATION AND HOW THE GUM MARGIN IS CLEANED WELL

You can see, therefore, that we must brush our top teeth and our bottom teeth, independently. Remember, also, that it is easy to clean the front facing surfaces of the teeth, but we must go inside and clean the inward facing surfaces of the teeth just as thoroughly as plaque accumulates there, too.

Sometimes, we have a crowded, rotated or mal-aligned tooth. When the teeth are not perfectly aligned, it would be easy to miss certain bits if we took long strokes when we are brushing. That is why **Tip number 2** is to take one or two teeth at a time and concentrate on brushing them really well, and then move the brush onto the next one or two teeth and brush those. It has been shown that as long as the brush is angled 45 degrees towards the gum margin, a side to side action is the most effective.

This tip allows you to concentrate correctly on where you are at the time and deal with any rotations or irregularities in the positions of the teeth. It also helps ensure that all the plaque is thoroughly removed. It is important to remember that what needs to be removed is the soft plaque so there is no need to brush too hard and scrub the teeth. If you do this, you will end up wearing down and damaging your teeth. That is why I always recommend a soft or medium brush.

Tip number 3 is to create a journey in your mouth that you stick to every day. This ensures that no part of the mouth is being missed because the brushing has been approached in a haphazard fashion. For example, I will brush the cheek side of my back (molar) teeth on the top left, two at a time, side to side with the angle of 45 degrees. I then methodically move around the cheek side surface of all of my top teeth, two at a time until I finally brush the teeth on the top right-hand side of my mouth. I then brush the biting surfaces of my top teeth, this time going from right to left. I then brush the inside surfaces of my top teeth all the way from left to right, again. Now that I am on the right, I move the brush down to brush the cheek side surfaces of my lower teeth, again, brushing them two at a time and moving my way round the mouth to the left. Then, I do the biting surfaces, and then finally I will brush the tongue side of my teeth again going from the right-hand side, all the way to the left.

The truth is it takes longer to explain or to read this technique than it does to actually do. And although it will take longer initially, I can comfortably and thoroughly brush my teeth within two minutes, so there is no reason why, after some practice, it will not be the same for you.

Within this book, I have put special free bonuses that I want you to have. In order to claim them, I want you to visit www.smilingdentist.co.uk where they are all posted.

Some of the bonuses have a limited availability so please do not delay. If you are one of the lucky first readers to take action and visit the site, you will be rewarded.

I will discuss all the bonuses throughout the book, so you will be reminded about them at the relevant times as the book progresses.

FREE BONUS

Visit www.smilingdentist.co.uk to see a short video on the brushing technique which shows you how best to brush your teeth.

Mistake 3: Not Flossing

Some patients are cleaning very well; you can see there is no plaque or bleeding gums when you look at the front or the inside surfaces of the teeth. However, I see a common problem when I examine the bit of the gum in between the teeth. I can see there is a lot of bleeding so it is obvious to me that the patient has not been effectively cleaning in between the teeth.

Unfortunately, brushing alone cannot clean these places well and so it is mandatory that the patient floss with some kind of aid to help them clean this area. Flossing is very effective, but it can be quite tricky and very time-consuming so there is also the option of using what is called an inter-dental brush.

Personally, I think inter-dental brushes are more effective. I find that the bristles tend to adapt very well to the part of the tooth that meets the neighbouring tooth (we call this part of the tooth the 'aproximal' surface). And, also the inter-dental brush tends to clean in between the teeth far quicker and easier. The brush shape looks like a very long, thin cylinder that you simply poke in between the teeth to dislodge any food or plaque that stagnates.

When people start cleaning in between their teeth, it is often the case that because the gums are inflamed in this area that they can bleed quite badly. The gums do stop bleeding and settle very well within the first 2 to 3 days as long as the cleaning is effective and maintained.

FREE BONUS

Please do look at the video on a brushing technique at www.smilingdentist.co.uk where a demonstration of interdental cleaning is shown.

Mistake 4: Not Getting Teeth Professionally Cleaned Often Enough

If plaque is allowed to stagnate for long enough in the mouth, then it will actually turn into a hard substance called 'calculus' or 'tartar'. There are minerals in the saliva and these minerals calcify the soft plaque. This turns it into the tartar which has a texture very similar to lime-scale.

The tartar is very rough and is often irregular. This allows plaque to adhere to it very easily. The more plaque that stagnates, the more will become calcified and so the more tartar will accumulate. This can become a vicious spiral with the amount of tartar growing every day.

Unfortunately, the tartar is quite hard and very tenacious and so it really is impossible for a patient to remove it at home. This is one of the main reasons why dentists and hygienists will clean your teeth professionally at your routine examinations. Thorough removal of the tarter really helps to ensure good gum health and prevention of serious gum disease.

If left for a long time, this tartar can also accumulate underneath the gum margin, deep on the root of the tooth. This is where it is most destructive to the bone and can rapidly increase bone loss. It is most important to remove this 'sub-gingival' tartar. However, it can often be quite uncomfortable so it might be necessary to have the teeth numbed to clean the teeth properly, and ensure that the procedure is comfortable.

Mistake 5: Using the Wrong Mouth Rinse

I have patients who will brush and floss and then use a mouth rinse containing 'Chlorhexidine'. Chlorhexidine does have some great advantages. It is proved to kill bacteria and so this mouthwash can be used as an antibacterial agent in the mouth. Chlorhexidine also has the advantage that it works over a long period of time. This is a property called 'substantivity'.

Although I recommend and prescribe this mouthwash for many situations, I do not normally recommend this as a daily rinse for my patients as it can stain the teeth if used over a long period of time. Chlorhexidine can cause a very bitter or metallic taste, as well. The rinse itself does not taste bad; in fact, it has quite a minty taste, but it alters the taste perception so everything that is tasted afterwards has a bitter or metallic taste.

The last problem with the mouthwash is that toothpaste has an ingredient called SLS (sodium-lauryl-sulphate) and if this SLS comes into contact with Chlorhexidine, it inactivates it. In essence, if people brush and then use this mouth rinse within 45 minutes of brushing (either before or after), it has no benefit at all.

There are many times when I recommend Chlorhexidine as a mouth rinse, particularly if patients have had surgery and cannot brush for a short period of time or if they have a bad infection. However, as a daily rinse I do not recommend it. I would normally direct patients towards something like Listerine which does not have the disadvantages as listed above and is safe to use daily.

As mentioned above, though, if patients can demonstrate that they can brush and floss effectively and have no inflammation in their mouths, then it is not necessary for them to use a mouth rinse at all.

Chapter 2

"Is Sugar Really That Bad?"

How and why sugar causes cavities and rots people's teeth, and how I can fix the holes in your teeth.

Causes of Decay

Sugars are simple carbohydrates. Dentists can categorise these into intrinsic and extrinsic sugars, but a simpler distinction is to separate them into the sugar that comes from fruit and milk, and all other sugars. For the purpose of this chapter, we are really dealing with the sugar that you find in all the other foods aside from fruit and milk. Dentists call these the non-milk extrinsic sugars or the NMEs. We have discussed earlier how there are many bacteria which reside in the mouth and many of these bacteria will ferment sugar (NME) that comes into the oral environment and turn it into acid.

Teeth are very hard because they have lots of mineral in their structure. The acid that the bacteria produce can dissolve the mineral. This process is called 'dental caries' or 'tooth decay'. As the mineral is dissolved from the tooth, certain changes happen. One change is that the tooth can become stained because as the mineral is removed from the tooth surface, it becomes slightly rougher. This means that the dietary products that cause stains (like tannins) that would not normally adhere to the teeth are able to do so. The teeth can also develop white spots and this is because minerals give the teeth their glass-like appearance, so removing the mineral alters the way that the tooth looks.

Normally the outside surface of the tooth (enamel) is very difficult to dissolve, so you normally only ever get a very small defect on the surface of the tooth. However, on the inside of the tooth is another substance called dentine. It is much easier for the dentine to lose its mineral, and so the decay process can happen much more rapidly on the inside of the tooth.

If a large amount of mineral is lost from the tooth substance, then it becomes dramatically weaker, often from the inside out. This is why patients can sometimes be eating on relatively soft food and suddenly the tooth will break or a hole or cavity will form.

As mentioned before, one of the main reasons why we ask patients to come regularly for dental examinations is that we can check if holes are forming within the tooth. This is also the reason why we regularly x-ray teeth. There are areas of the tooth which are particularly difficult to visually examine, but the decay in these areas does show up very clearly on x-rays. These same x-rays are also very good at examining patients' bone levels so they are used to help see if patients have gum problems, as well. That is why I now feel it is good practice to always take x-rays when I see patients for their first appointment.

Our inherent susceptibility to tooth decay is the biggest determining factor as to whether we will experience holes in our teeth or not. What I mean by this is that genetic factors are the most influential. Some peoples' teeth can be very densely packed with minerals whereas others will have very few minerals by comparison and they will be very loosely bound, and hence, easily dissolved. The other big factor is whether our saliva contains the type of bacteria which will rapidly cause decay or if it contains factors which help to protect the teeth.

Fundamentally, it is acid that dissolves the mineral in the tooth and when sugar enters the oral environment it is turned into acid by the bacteria in the saliva.

The pH scale measures how acidic something is. The mouth has to attain a certain level of acidity before the demineralisation associated with tooth decay happens. As soon as the body detects that the mouth is becoming too acidic it does its best to try and neutralise the acidity. Our saliva will increase so that it can wash away the sugary food and the acid that has been produced. Agents called buffers are also produced and these help to neutralise any acid that is there. The last way that the saliva can protect our teeth is by containing minerals. So when the mouth is acidic and the mineral is lost from the teeth, the mineral in the saliva can be used to re-mineralise and repair the teeth once again. Tooth decay happens when the net demineralisation is greater than the net re-mineralisation, i.e. the tooth is losing more mineral then it's gaining.

If the saliva inherently contains many of these protective factors and the salivary flow rate is very good, then it can also help to protect people against tooth decay. So you can see that somebody with very densely packed minerals in the tooth that also has many of the salivary protective agents is much less likely to be able to get tooth decay than somebody who doesn't. Conversely, if somebody has very 'soft' teeth with much less minerals that are loosely bound and also has many of the bacteria in the saliva that will promote decay rather than the factors that protect against it, then they will have to be very careful, otherwise their decay experience will be very high.

This is why I often see siblings who are exactly the same with respect to diet and teeth cleaning, and yet one will experience much more decay than the other one who may even have perfect teeth. I always try to explain this to patients, who I perceive have difficulty with decay, but I can only offer an explanation and it is not something that we can change. This is why dentists normally focus on the aspects that patients have some control over.

Overwhelmingly, the most important controllable factor is sugar intake. However, it is not the quantity of sugar that is as important as the frequency of intake. As discussed, the body does try to protect itself when sugar enters the mouth by releasing saliva that helps to neutralise the acid and repair the teeth. If a large amount of sugar is eaten in one sitting, then the mouth has a chance to neutralise that acid attack. However, if sugar is ingested frequently, then the oral environment will become acidic and an attempt will be made to neutralise it. If more sugar is consumed, it will become acidic again. Again, the body will attempt to neutralise the acid. And then there will be another acidic attack, etc. So it is apparent that the time that the mouth will be acidic is much longer when there are frequent intakes of sugar.

This means that the teeth are being demineralised for a much longer time than it is being re-mineralised or repaired. The mouth, therefore, becomes the perfect environment for the teeth to lose minerals until eventually, they rot from the inside out. This is why when I see patients who have many holes in their teeth, I discuss with them that it is apparent that we are going to have to do some operative treatments like fillings in order to repair the damage that has been done. However, it is much more important that we make some changes to the way that sugar is being consumed. It is imperative to cut down on the frequency of intake so that we do not allow the problem to persist, and hence cause more problems when I see them again in 6 months!

Good oral hygiene is also very important in preventing decay because if plaque can thoroughly be removed, then the bacteria that cause the decay are gone so it will offer some protection against it. However, I would always say that good oral hygiene is the most important factor in preventing gum disease, whereas diet and particularly sugar intake is really the most important factor when trying to prevent tooth decay.

There is an ingredient called fluoride which is also very important in helping to prevent tooth decay. Fluoride is a molecule which can be absorbed into the teeth, and when it is there, it helps to bind the minerals which make up the teeth much more tightly than the normal tooth structure does. You can find fluoride in practically all toothpaste and you can find it in specific mouth rinses, too. In some areas in the country, for instance in the West Midlands they add fluoride to water, again with the specific purpose of trying to lower rates of tooth decay, especially in children.

It is important to note, though, that too much fluoride can affect teeth, too. When children have their baby teeth, their adult teeth are still being formed. The cells that make these teeth are called ameloblasts and they are particularly sensitive cells. If people have too much fluoride at this age, it can affect these ameloblasts. When they lay the substance for the adult tooth down, they do not do it properly. This means that the appearance of the adult teeth can change, with brown or white spots.

This appearance is generally called 'Mottling', but if it is particularly caused by fluoride, it is called 'Fluorosis'. This is why it is important to use children's toothpaste on children's teeth because it has the correct dose of fluoride. It is also important to make sure that we do not put too much toothpaste on a child's toothbrush and make sure that they are supervised so we can make sure they are not simply eating all of the toothpaste.

Treatment of decay

As mentioned before, if patients have decay, especially in a number of teeth, the most important part of our treatment is to prevent further decay by assessing the diet and/or any other factors that may be causing the decay. We then make changes so that we can help prevent this from happening again.

'Fissure sealants' can also be placed on teeth as a preventative measure. They are like a varnish that is placed onto the tooth to seal the irregular biting surface and change the shape slightly. The rough biting surface can act as an excellent area for plaque and food to become trapped. This is why the most common area to find decay in a tooth is on the biting surface (in the areas we call the pits and fissures). By placing fissure sealants, we are able to modify the shape of the tooth so that it is smoother. This means plaque and food find it harder to stagnate, and hence it prevents decay from starting. The procedure is totally painless and requires no needle and no drilling. It is ideal for children and is often done for children as a preventative measure.

The other part of the treatment is the operative dentistry. This means the removal of the decay and the placement of fillings in any holes or cavities that are present for a variety of reasons so: 1) that patients can bite and chew without pain, 2) that the cavities can stop being food and plaque traps, 3) the teeth look presentable again and 4) that we can stop the spread of the decay.

If a patient has a decay cavity and it is full of bacteria, the bacteria will spread and make the hole bigger and bigger. That is why we need to remove all of the decay and the bacteria from the tooth so that we are left with a clean cavity which will not increase in size. We would normally numb the tooth so that the procedure is not painful. This would most likely involve a local anaesthetic injection. (There will be more on anaesthesia in Chapter 10.) At this point, it is important to fill the tooth again so that we do not have a hole that can act as a trap for food and plaque that can stagnate once more.

The filling allows us to build the tooth back up to the correct size and shape so that we are able to use it as an effective chewing platform and also so that it looks correct. Traditionally in the back teeth, this has been done with a metal filling for many years but it is now much more common for us to use the tooth coloured fillings which used to be much more common in the front teeth. Tooth coloured fillings have two main advantages: one is obviously the appearance of a tooth so anyone looking into your mouth when conversing with you will be unaware that you have had decay in your teeth or that you have had it treated. The other big advantage is that white fillings are bonded or glued into the teeth. This is not critical in keeping the filling in the tooth because metal fillings which are not glued in do not normally fall out. The big advantage comes when you have a large cavity because often, what is left of the tooth, can be very thin and fragile walls.

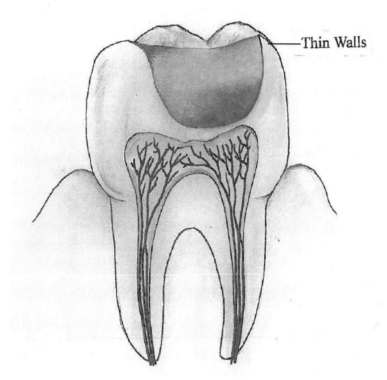

Thin Walls

ILLUSTRATION OF A LARGE CAVITY SHOWING HOW THIN THE WALLS
OF TOOTH CAN BE AFTER THE DECAY HAS BEEN REMOVED

If you are able to bond the filling, then essentially the thin wall is bonded to the filling which is again bonded to the other thin wall. When everything is bonded together like this, it makes the whole structure much stronger.

If decay has spread so much, you can find it spreads into the nerve in the tooth

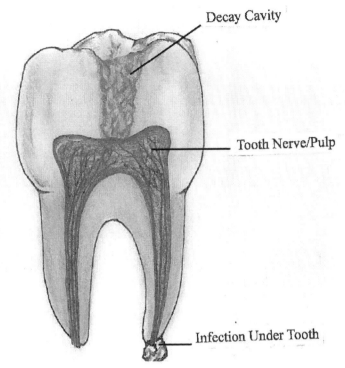

Decay Cavity

Tooth Nerve/Pulp

Infection Under Tooth

ILLUSTRATION OF THE CROSS-SECTION OF A TOOTH SHOWING
TOOTH DECAY THAT HAS SPREAD INTO THE NERVE AND CAUSED
INFECTION.

This is the most common cause of toothache. Unfortunately, if the situation has been allowed to get this bad, than normally simply filling the tooth is not enough. If the decay is allowed to get into the nerve, the same bacteria that cause the decay also cause the nerve to become inflamed or irritated. If we remove the decay and simply place a filling in the tooth, then the irritated and inflamed nerve will continue to cause pain and this can also lead to an infection or an abscess around the tooth. That is why, if there is pain in the teeth, a different treatment option is needed. At this point, there are really only two choices. One is to fully remove the tooth; i.e. an extraction, and the other option is to do root canal treatment. (This will be explained further in the next chapter.)

Another big danger if the decay is allowed to spread is that it will spread very deep into the root of the tooth. If this happens and the decay is removed, the margin of the restoration (where the tooth and filling meet) will be too deep under the gum on the root of the tooth. At this point, it is impossible to place a filling that will adequately seal the tooth and prevent further decay. If the seal is not obtained, bacteria are able to get back into the tooth and this is when the decay can start again. This is one of the few times when patients have to be told that the only option is to remove the tooth.

There are times when cavities in the teeth can be very, very big and when the decay is removed there is so little tooth left that it is too weak to adequately retain a filling. When this happens, there is the option of placing a crown on the tooth. The crown is a different type of restoration and is far stronger than a filling.

Essentially, it is like a crash helmet for the tooth. To give you an idea it is like a hat that is around 1 mm thick all the way round. The tooth is smoothed down 1 mm all the way around so that it can provide room for the crown. This means that when the crown is fitted onto the tooth, the tooth goes back to being the correct size and shape that it was at the start and does not interfere in the bite.

Crowns are custom-made for teeth. The procedure involves smoothing down the tooth and then making an impression of the teeth. The impression of the teeth is sent to a laboratory and the model of the teeth is made. The crown is made to fit very accurately on the model of the patient's teeth and afterwards, that crown is sent back to the dentist. A second appointment for the patient is made when the crown is ready and the crown is fitted onto the tooth. The crown often needs some slight adjustment, but it is a very good fit and usually the best and most long lasting restoration we can provide.

Chapter 3

"I Have a Toothache! What Should I Do?"

From sensitive teeth to a raging toothache, I will explain what you need to do.

Tooth anatomy

Teeth are made up of three layers. On the outside there is a very hard substance called enamel. The enamel has no sensation, whatsoever, that is why we are able to drill into enamel or polish the enamel without using any anaesthetic knowing there will be no pain at all. Inside the enamel is a layer called dentine. It is softer than enamel, though quite hard in its own right. The dentine does have some sensation and if we were to drill into it or if the dentine layer became exposed and subjected to cold or hot, you would certainly feel that because the sensation would be conveyed through the third layer of the tooth: the 'dental pulp' or the nerve. Incidentally, the nerve in the tooth can only express pain. It is a very primitive nerve with only pain fibres; it cannot tell the brain anything about where it is.

When you touch your hand, you can tell exactly where you have been touched. If you are touched close to your thumb, your brain can very accurately detect this. Likewise, if you have been touched close to your little finger, the brain is able to distinguish this. The acute perception of touch is called 'proprioception'. The nerve in the tooth has no proprioceptive fibres, whereas the areas surrounding the tooth do. I will explain later why this is an important distinction.

Inside the dentine of the tooth resides the nerve. We, as dentists actually call it the 'Dental Pulp' because it is a very complicated network of nerves and blood vessels all intertwined. Within the pulpal mass are also cells which are able to lay down new tooth structure.

Whenever there is pain in the tooth, it is caused either because there is some kind of exposure which means that the dentine is exposed to the oral environment, or it means that the nerve in the tooth is dying or the nerve has died. This means that the nerve is transmitting pain signals to the brain or there is an infection surrounding the tooth and that is causing the sensation of pain to be conveyed to the brain.

I should make it clear at this point that this chapter is only really concerned with pain which is coming from the teeth and the surrounding structures. There are many other causes of pain in the mouth, some of which are very complicated to diagnose and these are probably beyond the scope of this book.

Sensitive/exposed dentine

The dentine from the tooth can be exposed for a number of reasons. The tooth can become decayed and a cavity can form and this exposes the inside of the tooth. The tooth can be damaged by hard food or by trauma of some kind. If the tooth fractures, it can also cause the dentine to be exposed. Gum around the tooth can shrink away or recede and this can expose dentine around the neck of the tooth. If patients grind their teeth they can also cause damage to the necks of the teeth. These are called abfraction lesions.

There is some debate amongst dentists as to why dentine is sensitive and why, if exposed, the dentine causes pain in the teeth. If you look at the dentine under a microscope, you see that it has many tiny little tubes or tubules in it. These tubules go from the surface, where the dentine meets the enamel, all the way into the middle of the tooth where the nerve is. These tubules are filled with fluid.

Most dentists agree that it is the movement of this fluid that causes the pain in the nerve. That is why the most common thing that causes sensitivity are things that can have an effect on fluid like heat which can expand the fluid, cold which can contract it, and sugar which can move the fluid through a process known as osmosis.

The best treatment for sensitivity of this kind is to try to fill and block the entrance to those tubules. If there is a large cavity in the tooth, then doing a filling is, practically speaking, the best way to do that. But if, for instance, with gum recession there is no actual cavity of any size, then I actually advise the patient against a filling. Because the cavity is so small and thin, any filling placed to fill in this cavity will be far too small and weak and will probably break and fallout very quickly.

There are however many 'sensitive' toothpastes on the market and I find some of these to be very effective. I tend to recommend 'Sensodyne Repair and Protect' as it has an ingredient which can very effectively lay it self down in the tubules and block them. I generally have very good feedback from my patients about how their sensitivity decreases dramatically when they use this toothpaste properly. Unfortunately, I do not think the manufacturers make a point enough about how to use it and that's why I end up speaking to all of my patients about the specifics of this as outlined below.

The sensitive toothpaste can be used in one of two ways:

If the sensitivity is generalised (so it is affecting more than one of the teeth often in different areas in the mouth), I tend to ask my patients to use it as a toothpaste. However, the key thing here is to brush with the toothpaste as normal but then to spit the excess out but not rinse the mouth. A residue must be left so that it is able to coat the teeth, penetrate into the dentine tubules, and block them. If the mouth is rinsed, the residue will be washed away and the toothpaste will be useless in helping with the sensitivity.

The other way it can be used is especially beneficial if the sensitivity is localised; say for instance, there are only one or two particular teeth which are sensitive. In this case, I instruct patients to brush with whichever toothpaste they prefer using to clean their teeth, and then after they have rinsed their mouth, they use the sensitive toothpaste like an ointment. They take some on their finger and smear it onto the tooth where the sensitivity is and just leave the paste there. Normally, I advise patients to do this at night time so that they can go to sleep with the sensitive toothpaste in place to give the maximum benefit.

FREE BONUS

Visit the book website www.smilingdentist.co.uk to request a goody bag containing Sensodyne samples

Cracked cusp syndrome

Teeth can break when being used and sometimes the fracture is not complete. What I mean is that often when the tooth breaks, part of it will come away completely and this is what we call a complete fracture. Other times, a crack will appear or start, but nothing will break away. When this happens, it can be a real problem to diagnose. If the fracture line is very small, it can be almost impossible to detect. Even when an x-ray is taken, the fracture has to be in exactly the right place for it to appear on the x-ray.

The cusp of the tooth is the sharp bit on the biting surface that protrudes slightly from the tooth.

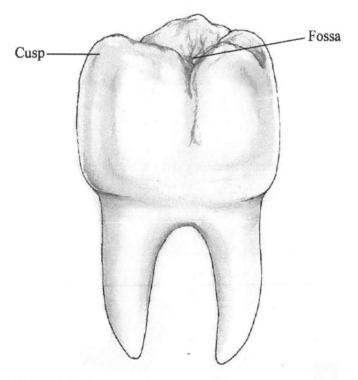

ILLUSTRATION OF A TOOTH SHOWING THE CUSPS AND FOSSAE

When a cusp fractures in this way, it will cause a pain when the tooth is being bitten on and it can also cause sensitivity in the tooth. The reason is because when the tooth is loaded, the fractured part of it will flex and this movement causes pain.

The other problem is that when the fracture appears, the seal of the tooth is compromised so bacteria can potentially get into the nerve in the tooth. This can cause the nerve to die in much the same way as it would if there was very deep decay in the tooth.

The correct treatment is determined by how large the fracture is. If it is very small, it can be treated with a filling. I would always recommend a bonded filling because that helps to strengthen the tooth that is left. This can be important because although the main fracture is removed when drilling the tooth for the filling, there may be other small fractures which have not really started yet. But bonding the filling can prevent propagation of those fractures. If the nerve has been involved, it is possible to start getting symptoms of sensitivity with hot and cold.

You normally would not expect these symptoms because if it is a tooth fracture, you only really expect pain when loading the tooth. This can complicate the diagnosis, but if the nerve is involved, often root canal treatment is necessary in addition to any treatment to try and remove the fracture and strengthen and protect the tooth. Root canal treatment will be discussed later in this chapter.

If the fracture is larger and the tooth is significantly weakened, it may need a crown. As discussed in the previous chapter, crowns are stronger restorations and act as a 'crash helmet for the tooth'. This will help to protect the remaining tooth structure, even if it is cracked and compromised to some extent.

The difficulty in treating these cases is being able to detect the extent of the fracture because it is often not obvious at all. The magnitude of the pain does not give any clue because sometimes very painful fractures can be small and less painful fractures can be big. It is important for the patient to understand that there may be a number of visits worth of treatment before the correct specific diagnosis can be made and the correct treatment can be provided.

Pulpitis

Fillings are put into a very hostile environment bathed constantly with saliva and subject to cyclic loading when chewing, so it is not surprising that as time goes by they do breakdown. If they break down around the margin i.e. the point where the filling meets the tooth, the seal can be compromised and the filling will begin to leak. Only a microscopic gap is needed before bacteria can enter and find their way underneath the filling. These bacteria can then get in through the dentine tubules to the nerve in the tooth and cause inflammation or irritation. This can cause pain most notably sensitivity with hot or cold. The best way to treat this is to replace the filling because very often when the seal is re-established, the nerve has a chance to calm down and the sensitivity reduces. This is called 'reversible pulpitis'.

However, in my experience it is less common to get the nerve to resolve if it is inflamed; and the exact state that the nerve is in plays a massive part in determining whether it will get better or not. If the inflammation or irritation in the nerve has gone past a certain point, then whatever we do, the nerve will not resolve. If this happens, we must remove the nerve in order to ensure that the tooth gets better and the pain stops.

Inflammation is a normal body process and one that is designed to help us to repair ourselves after we have been damaged in some way. Damage is usually caused by chemical, burn, irritant, trauma or infection. Inflammation is the process by which the body directs blood flow to the area so that the cells within the blood can help to heal and repair, or fight off cells that are not meant to be there, like in the process of infection.

A good example is if you bang yourself on the arm. The tissue swells and feels tender. That bump you get is caused by inflammation. It is a very helpful process and one that is integral to our survival. However, in the tooth, this is not helpful. The problem is that we have soft tissue surrounded by a wall of hard tissue, i.e. the nerve of the tooth encased in the dentine of the tooth. Also, we have one communication of blood supply in and out which is at the bottom of the root (the apex).

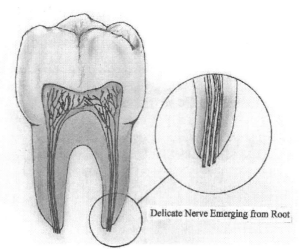

Delicate Nerve Emerging from Root

ILLUSTRATION OF A TOOTH WITH THE NERVE EMERGING OUT OF THE ROOT APEX

When swelling happens in the nerve of the teeth, pressure builds up which cannot escape and this is why you experience intense pain. This pain we know as a toothache. The other problem is that at the bottom of the root of the tooth, where the pulp tissue enters the tooth, the pressure increase constricts the vessels so that no nutrients can get into the pulp and eventually the nerve dies. This painful process is made worse by the fact that this constriction also means that no painkillers, that are taken and go into the bloodstream, can be delivered into the nerve where it could really help with the inflammation.

There are really only two options when this happens: one is that the tooth must be removed or we must get into the nerve to make access and allow the pressure to drop. The second is the procedure that we would do in the first stage of root canal treatment.

We discussed earlier in this chapter how the type of nerve that we have in the pulp is primitive and how it is unable to convey any sensation of where it is, i.e. proprioception. It is only able to tell the brain that there is pain. Often, when you have this kind of toothache, you definitely know it is painful, but it is almost impossible for the brain to exactly tell which tooth it is happening in.

Sometimes, the brain can mistake where the sensation is coming from and it will be convinced that the pain is coming from a bottom tooth when actually it is coming from the top tooth. This can also be a very challenging diagnosis to make, but it is helpful to the dentist because it allows him/her to tell from the patient's history exactly what is going on in the nerve. When a patient has this pain from pulpitis, it normally causes sensitivity with hot food and drink and also variable sensitivity to cold.

The art of diagnosing comes from knowing that everybody's reaction to the same pathology can be different and also knowing that the stage in which you see somebody, within the disease process, can affect the way that they present. I make this point because with some people hot will be very painful and cold will also be very painful, whereas, with others, hot will be painful but cold will be quite soothing. I have also seen a few patients with pulpitis who will put heat packs on the teeth in order to soothe the pain even though you would expect heat to be the worst thing for a tooth with pulpitis.

The important distinction is that after hot or cold food or drink has been consumed, the pain lasts for some time after heat/cold has been removed. When this pulpitis gets bad there can also be spontaneous pain, i.e. pain without any hot or cold stimulus. Unfortunately, night-time is a common time for the pain and patients routinely report getting this kind of pain.

As the nerve starts to die, it becomes necrotic which means that the nerve tissue starts to rot inside the tooth. It becomes a wonderful medium for bacteria to colonise and once the bacteria are in, they can multiply quite rapidly.

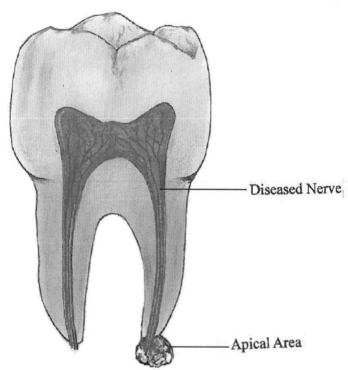

Diseased Nerve

Apical Area

ILLUSTRATION OF A DISEASED TOOTH WITH APICAL AREA (ROOT TIP INFECTION)

Tooth Abscesses

When bacteria find a way out of the end of the root of the tooth, the 'root apex', they can form an abscess around the bottom of the tooth. The abscess can be very fast growing and cause lots of pain (acute dental abscess), or it can be very slow growing and virtually painless (chronic dental abscess). It is important to note that even these chronic painless abscesses can become infected by different bacteria and if this happens they will turn into a particularly nasty acute abscess. The big problem with the chronic abscess is that it eats away at the bone and this can sometimes affect other teeth.

The pain and the swelling is now affecting the areas surrounding the tooth (the periodontal tissues); and these tissues do have proprioceptive fibres so they can tell the brain exactly where they are. This means that it is relatively easy for the patient to point to the tooth and say, "This is the one that hurts".

Sometimes the tooth can be raised slightly by the swelling underneath it so it will often feel very painful to bite on the tooth because it is slightly higher in the bite. Sometimes because the tissue is spongy around the infection, the tooth can feel a little bit wobbly, as well. Normally, if the nerve has fully died and there is just a big abscess around the tooth, then there is no sensitivity with hot and cold because the nerve in the tooth has gone and, therefore, it is unable to convey that sensation to the brain.

However, you can see that one process often flows into another so it is possible to have a tooth which has more than one root, and hence more than one nerve. If one nerve is in the process of dying, yet another one is dead, it will be possible to get a mixture of the symptoms outlined above. Therefore the tooth would be very sensitive with hot and cold, but also it will be clear which tooth is causing the pain. If the tooth is tapped, it will also be very painful.

You can see how important it is for a dentist to ask lots of questions about the nature of the pain when somebody attends with a toothache, because in some instances, it is possible to arrive at a diagnosis almost virtually from the history alone. Sometimes, however, the history is a little bit confusing and does not fall neatly into a single category. Thus, it is always important for the dentist to look very carefully at the teeth to see if there are any clues and also to take some radiographs to help assess whether there are any changes that have happened inside the tooth or around the roots which cannot be seen with the naked eye. This, along with some specific tests, can really help the dentist to get a picture of what is happening and that is the first step in planning the treatment that can rectify the pain.

It is also important to note that these processes do not always happen painfully. Nerves can die silently and sometimes patients have an abscess around the tooth without experiencing any pain from pulpitis; while sometimes patients present no pain and it is only when I take an x-ray, perhaps for another reason, that we can see that there is a large chronic abscess around the tooth.

Treatment for Dental Nerve Pain

If the nerve has died or is in the process of dying then, as touched on earlier, one way or another we need to remove that nerve from the mouth. There are only two options for doing this:

1) If we wish to save the tooth, then we have to do a procedure called root canal treatment. This involves making a hole in the top of the tooth so that we can find the nerve. The nerve is cleaned out and the inside of the tooth is disinfected so that all the bacteria are killed. The space that the nerve used to occupy needs to be filled and the root canal is all sealed back up again.

Root Filling Material Being Placed

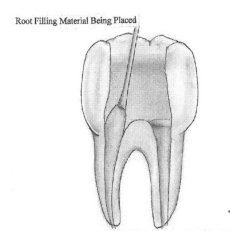

ILLUS-
TRATION
OF A
TOOTH
WITH A
ROOT
CANAL
FILLING
BEING
PLACED

Root Filling in Place Sealing the Root Canal Space

Sometimes we are able to put a filling back onto the tooth where we have filled the root canal, but other times the tooth is so badly broken down that we need to put a crown on the tooth. It is more common for the tooth to require a crown, especially with the back teeth, because the back teeth do come under much higher forces. This means that it is easier for the weakened root-treated tooth to break, if the tooth is not reinforced.

Most patients ask me when they hear me planning root canal treatment, 'is it painful?' The honest answer is that it depends. If the nerve is dead and there is an abscess around the tooth, the root canal treatment is absolutely painless as there is no longer any nerve in the tooth to convey the pain to the brain.

Whether the nerve is still alive in the tooth or dead, I would administer anaesthetic to numb the tooth. This means that the majority of times there is no feeling. But I do always warn that there could be slight pain because there are a very few cases where the pressure build-up in the nerve is so high that it is difficult to obtain anaesthesia (complete numbness). When this happens, it is clear that the anaesthetic has worked because all the surrounding tissues are numb. But when we start to make the access into the tooth, there is definitely some feeling.

However, it is transient because as soon as we get into the nerve and release the pressure, the tooth numbs-up very nicely and we are able to continue and complete the procedure without there being any pain.

Doing proper root canal treatment does take time and skill. The advantages of root canal treatment are that you can keep the tooth, but the procedure takes longer and is inevitably more costly than the alternative. The other thing to note is that root canal treatment is not 100% successful, and even in the best possible hands there will be times where it will fail.

2) The only alternative option is to take the painful tooth out. This involves numbing the tooth and essentially pushing on the tooth in a way that it does not like, until it starts to wobble and eventually comes out.

Again, this is not a painful procedure because of the numbing, but there is a lot of pushing involved. Removing a tooth does have its advantages; it is quicker than doing the root canal treatment and normally simpler. Thus, the cost involved is normally less. However when a tooth is removed it does leave a gap and sometimes it can cost more money to fill that gap in. Often, it is appropriate to leave a gap, but important for the patient to know that often the teeth surrounding the gap can move and this can sometimes have consequences for the bite and potentially for any future plans to fill the gap. That is why it is often prudent to plan replacement of teeth soon after they are removed.

Gum abscesses

The last major reason for pain from the teeth comes from particularly bad gums. Sometimes the bacteria that cause gum disease can also cause abscesses around the teeth. If one is particularly prone to getting abscesses from gum origin, it could be that there is some underlying medical condition that needs investigating and treating. I must be clear that this is not always the case, but sometimes it can be a sign that diabetes or impaired immune function (which means that the body's defence cells are not working properly) is present. If it has not been diagnosed it may be worth going to see a general medical practitioner so that tests can be run just, so that they can rule it out.

Gum abscesses are normally treated by providing antibiotics, followed by cleaning the area thoroughly. This procedure requires numbing the tooth first so that the root of the tooth can be cleaned as this procedure would be uncomfortable if the area was not numbed first.

Chapter 4

"Why Does My Breath Smell?"

I will show you how to treat this common problem which can have serious social con-sequences.

Bad breath or 'Halitosis' is a common condition which affects many people at one time or another. It is usually caused by eating something pungent like garlic or onions. This is because certain sulphur containing compounds are released by these foods so they linger in the mouth. Therefore, the smell is released directly from the mouth. However, when these foods are eaten, they are metabolised and find their way into the bloodstream.

When the blood passes to the lungs, as it circulates around the body, the molecules containing the pungent sulphides pass from the blood, through the lungs, to the air and evaporate and come out in your breath. This is why one can brush his/her teeth and use mouth rinse and also chew gum, but the smell will still emanate for some time afterwards.

Chronic bad breath is less common and normally does necessitate some investigation.

Overwhelmingly, the most common causes of bad breath come from the mouth although there are sometimes causes which originate in the stomach or lower down in the gut.

Halitosis is most commonly caused by a build-up of tartar and plaque in the mouth causing the gums to be inflamed. The inflamed and swollen gums can harbour more plaque and sometimes food can then get trapped, in between the teeth and gums, and as the food rots and the bacteria reside, it can cause a bad taste and often a bad smell.

If this is the cause, the treatment of choice is to have a thorough professional cleaning and some modification in home cleaning to prevent the repeat build-up of plaque and tartar.

The optimum technique for brushing the teeth has been outlined in Chapter 1. A video of this technique is a special bonus which can be seen on the website www.smilingdentist.co.uk.

Sometimes there is a particular area in the mouth that traps food and this can also cause a bad smell. If, after meals, food is able to stay in the mouth then, this too, can stagnate and rot and hence a bad smell is released. The cause normally needs some investigation, too. Sometimes it can be because the teeth are malaligned or it could be because of a cavity that formed in a tooth or maybe a filling that is failing and allowing food to lodge underneath it.

Sometimes wisdom teeth can also cause food trapping and this will be covered more in Chapter 8. It is important that a thorough examination is done so that the correct cause of the bad smell is identified before it can be eliminated.

The chronic, slow-growing infections mentioned in the last chapter can also be a cause of bad taste and bad smell. Sometimes the infected liquid (containing lots of bacteria) can drain out by the side of the tooth or higher in the gum. This liquid tastes bad and can create a very bad smell.

Mouth rinse can be very helpful when somebody suffers with halitosis. I will always advise an effective daily rinse for someone with halitosis so I would probably suggest that something containing chlorhexidine is not the ideal option for the reasons outlined in chapter 1. I would normally suggest something like Listerine as a good option to help freshen breath.

FREE BONUS

Visit the book website www.smilingdentist.co.uk where you can request a free goody bag with mouth rinse, toothpaste and other oral hygiene aids.

One good tip is to brush the tongue when brushing the teeth. Although generally the skin in the mouth sheds periodically, so has some element of self-cleansing, the cells on the tongue can get trapped there for some time. As these cells breakdown and rot, they can also release a bad smell. This is why it is advisable to brush the tongue to remove these cells and facilitate the shedding. There is a specific instrument called a 'tongue scraper' that has been designed for this purpose and it can also be very good to use.

If all potential dental causes have been eliminated, i.e. all fillings done, cleaning done effectively, and also modifications have been made to the home care regime of brushing, flossing, and using a mouth rinse; and if there is still a bad smell coming from the mouth then it would be advisable to seek the help of the general medical practitioner who would be able to do certain investigations to eliminate causes that may arise from the stomach. Normally, however, if you approach a medical doctor first they will advise you to seek the help of the dentist to eliminate any potential dental causes because they also know that oral causes are, by far and away, the most common.

Chapter 5

"My Teeth Are Too Dark. What Can I Do About Them?"

How you can safely whiten your teeth and how not to do it.

Teeth darken most commonly because of molecules that are present in food and drink which can stain the teeth. The most common one that we come across is tannin which is abundant in tea, coffee, and red wine. The other very common reason is smoking where tar deposits are left on the teeth as the smoke enters the mouth and stays within the mouth before it is exhaled.

The appearance of teeth can also be changed by illnesses or medicines that could have affected the body at the time when the teeth are being formed.

Adult teeth develop deep in the gum when we still have our baby teeth in our mouths. If you have an illness like measles or take medicines like tetracycline antibiotics, they can affect the very sensitive cells called ameloblasts and odontoblasts which are responsible for laying down the enamel and dentine of the tooth. This can cause the tooth to look very dark and alter the appearance significantly. Excessive fluoride can cause a similar effect as discussed in Chapter 2.

Staining can be intrinsic (which means that it is held within the tooth structure) or extrinsic (which means it sits on top of the surface of the tooth). Most commonly the stain is a mixture of both. The type of stain will affect the treatment plan. If it is mainly extrinsic staining, cleaning and polishing will be very effective and you will see a massive change. If however the staining is intrinsic, and therefore held within the tooth structure, then a dentist could clean and polish the tooth all day and would not be able to remove this stain. When this happens, we must use different techniques that are able to penetrate within the tooth.

The most common is called 'Tooth Whitening'. This involves the use of a gel which is made up of either carbamide peroxide or hydrogen peroxide. Both of these gels are able to penetrate deep within the tooth and, when they do, they release oxygen which helps to remove the stain particles which bubble up and release it from the tooth. This removal of stains which has accumulated over many years actually makes the tooth, and hence the smile, look considerably whiter.

The beauty of whitening is that it causes no damage to the enamel or the dentine. Even at a microscopic level, you cannot tell the difference between a tooth that has been whitened and tooth that has not been. That is why it is one of my favourite dental treatments to do.

The only real downside with whitening is that it is common for the teeth to feel sensitive during or after the whitening treatment. This is happening less with new whitening techniques, especially when an ingredient is added to the whitening gel called ACP (amorphous calcium phosphate) which acts as a soothing gel and reduces the sensitivity.

Even if the teeth do become sensitive during treatment, they will always go back to being how they were before the treatment started. If there was no sensitivity before whitening, there will be no sensitivity after, and if there was some sensitivity before, it will go back to being at the same level.

There are two main ways to whiten teeth. There is **Home Whitening** or the 'tray method' which involves making moulds of teeth so that clear plastic trays can be made which fit onto the teeth very intimately. These trays fit the teeth very well. The whitening gel can be put into these trays and then placed in the mouth. These trays hold the gel against the teeth for long enough for them to do their job. Because they are very well-fitting, the gel does not escape from the trays. This is important because the peroxide in the gel can irritate the gums quite severely and will cause a chemical burn.

The process of filling the trays and wearing them for a given time is repeated every day for (normally) a two week period. The end result over this time is normally very good, as long as the trays have been worn for the correct amount of time.

One big advantage of this method is that if the trays are kept safe, then more gel can always be purchased relatively inexpensively, so that top up whitening can be done at a later date.

It is inevitable that staining from the diet will start to diminish the whiteness of the teeth again. It is important for you to be aware of this before the whitening treatment is done and a good idea for us to be able to do something like the 'top-up whitening' so that we can protect the results over the long term

The other main way that teeth can be whitened is by doing a whitening procedure in the surgery (**In-surgery whitening**). Normally around a two hour slot is booked and at the start of the treatment all of the gums and lips are isolated away from the teeth so that gel cannot go anywhere that it is not meant to. Then the gel is applied to the teeth and there is normally some activation of the gel either by light or by heat. The idea is that this activation speeds up the whitening process so that in the two hours in surgery, you get a far superior result when compared with two hours simply wearing trays at home. It used to be that the in-surgery whitening would use a much stronger gel, and because its use was supervised by a dentist, it was safe to do. However, the European Union regulations changed and that meant that the strong whitening gel that dentists used to use was outlawed.

This means that the gel used when making the trays and the gel used in surgery is normally off a similar concentration, and hence it really is the activation of the gel that is important when we are doing the whitening in surgery now.

The best results are obtained by using a combination approach which includes whitening the teeth in surgery and also providing trays which are used for whitening on the days immediately prior to, or after the in-surgery session. Some systems will do the whitening in surgery first and others do it at the end; and there is very little evidence to suggest that one method is better than the other.

There is another less common but very neat way of delivering of whitening gel to the tooth surface. This is via the use of the strip. It is a little bit like a clear sticking plaster that you apply to your teeth and it has whitening gel in it. It tends to be considerably cheaper than the tray whitening and the in-surgery whitening; and although many dentists may not like to admit it, this method can actually yield very good results. I really like this method because I feel it allows whitening to be accessible to many more patients than it was before.

Another common and cheap method of whitening the teeth that I have come across is with the use of whitening toothpastes. This is one method I do have to caution patients about. There are two methods by which whitening toothpastes work. One is by adding peroxide to the toothpaste, and that is the same ingredient that is in whitening gel. The other way is to add abrasive particles, normally silica to the toothpaste. The problem is that peroxide normally needs a long time to work when touching the teeth so there may only be limited benefit. The peroxide containing toothpaste may not be in contact with the tooth for long enough for it to provide any real benefit.

I do have some reservations with the abrasive toothpastes, because with daily use, they will significantly wear down the enamel on your teeth. Prolonged use can damage the tooth surface. And because the brightness of the tooth comes from the enamel, if it is worn away, the tooth will look darker and even professional whitening will not be able to whiten it very well. I normally advise patients to exercise some caution when using abrasive toothpaste. I think it is acceptable to use, but probably used more safely on a weekly basis rather than daily.

Sometimes patients come to me with one or two teeth that are particularly dark when compared to their other teeth. There are a number of ways to treat this, but one of my favourite ways is to do what we call 'inside-outside whitening'. Very commonly, if one tooth is dark it means that the nerve in the tooth has died and the dark products that are released by the dying nerve can start to travel through the tooth and make it look dark. The dentist would normally remove the nerve from the tooth and do a procedure called root canal treatment (Chapter 3) and then leave a hole in the back of the tooth. If we then do whitening with the trays as described above, the gel is able to surround the tooth from the outside as it normally would, but it can also get into the hole and whiten from within. This dramatically speeds up the whitening in the dark tooth so it catches up with the other teeth and very soon the colours of the teeth all match once again.

Dark teeth can also be covered with restorations like veneers and crowns. And indeed, if the shape or position of the tooth is also incorrect or if you want to improve the relative teeth proportions, I would normally recommend dental veneers as the treatment of choice. The veneers can be made to be very bright, and hence whitening the teeth that are going to be veneered is often unnecessary.

We will discuss veneers in much greater detail in the next chapter.

Chapter 6

"I Don't Like My Smile. What Can I Do?"

Colour, shape, size, crooked? I can show
you how to fix it all.

Smiles are so important! They are the focal point, right in the middle of the face. A smile conveys so much emotion. People who are confident with their smile convey this happiness to others. Studies show that nice smiles are linked with success, wealth, and improved social status. And it goes without saying, that a nice smile is more attractive to the opposite (or the same) sex!

People who do not have nice smiles may not be as confident when smiling, and will often be mistaken as being miserable, grumpy, angry or guarded. There are also many connotations linked with having 'ugly' teeth like being dirty or stupid. I look at smiles all the time and I very rarely see ugly smiles in successful people, especially in the media spotlight. It is becoming increasingly important to have a nice smile and is becoming much less socially acceptable to have an unattractive smile.

So what is a nice smile; how does one define it?

Before I became a dentist I knew when a smile was nice. When I speak to non-dentists, it is clear that people can pick up on what is a nice and what is not a nice smile. But it has taken me years of training to 'diagnose' an unattractive smile and recognise the elements that make a smile look nice and hence pick up the things that deviate from a perfect smile.

I want to discuss the secrets now so that you will become much more aware of what makes a smile look nice. I think you will be able to have some fun looking at the glossy magazines, looking at people who have had smile makeovers and deciding if they have been done well or not!

Most of the time, the brain picks up on an overall impression of a smile and will only really consciously know that it looks nice or that it doesn't look nice. Smiles that don't look nice will have broken one of the following cardinal rules:

Smiles need to be symmetrical, have good proportions, and they must fit into the face properly. Furthermore, the teeth cannot be too crooked.

Smiles that look great will adhere to all of the above and will also look better because the teeth are perfectly straight and because they are white. I will go into a little bit of detail about each of these elements now.

Symmetry

The teeth on the left-hand side should look the same as the teeth on the right. If they do not, the eyes will pick up that there is an imbalance in the way that the smile looks and register that the smile does not look attractive. The critical teeth in providing symmetry are the two big front teeth, the central incisors. If these two teeth look different then we have a big problem. As the teeth go further back, if the corresponding tooth on the other side looks different it is much more forgivable because it is much harder for the eye to pick up on that discrepancy. This is why it is common for cosmetic dentists to provide pairs of veneers at the very front of the mouth to avoid the discrepancy that would be inherent if only a single front tooth had to be done. This is because it is often easy to distinguish the subtle differences between a veneer and a natural tooth if the two teeth are side-by-side. Incidentally, it is not always necessary to provide the front teeth restorations as a pair. However it can be very difficult to get the restorations looking just right

Another problem can occur if the centre-line is off. This means that ideally you would like the centre-line (where the front two teeth meet) to be lined up with the midline of the face. However, this is not a 'deal breaker' and very often you do see people walking around with the dental centre-line which has shifted bodily left or right, and often you do not notice.

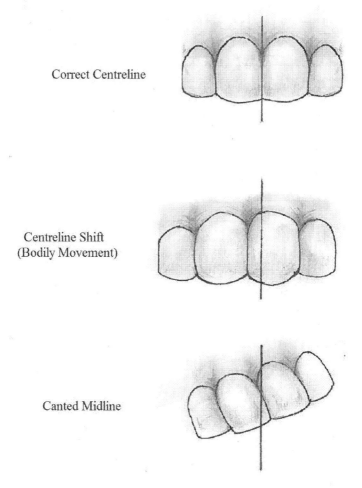

Correct Centreline

Centreline Shift
(Bodily Movement)

Canted Midline

ILLUSTRATION SHOWING HOW SMILES CAN APPEAR WHEN MEAS-
URED AGAINST THE MIDLINE OF THE FACE

A very famous example of someone with a smile like this is Tom Cruise who has only one central incisor which is right in the middle and yet people always talk about how great Tom Cruise's smile is (and it is great!). However if the centre line is not straight, i.e. if it is diagonal or angled (the term we use is canted), then the eye will pick that up very quickly and the smile will not look right at all.

Proportions

Proportions are also very important.

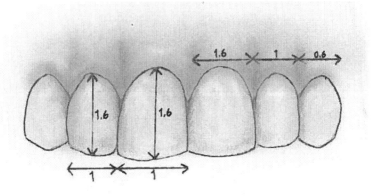

Golden Proportion

ILLUSTRATION OF A SMILE SHOWING WHERE GOLDEN PROPORTION IS SEEN

This includes the proportions of the teeth themselves with regard to their height and width but also the proportions of one tooth to another (specifically the proportions of the teeth that you see when looking at the smile). There is beautiful guide called 'Golden Proportion' which is the most attractive proportion and is one that we see commonly in everyday life. A normal A4 piece of paper has the height to width ratio that is in golden proportion. It appears in nature all the time; and as a result, it has been picked up and copied when manufacturing to make objects appear more attractive to our eyes. The proportion is 0.6:1 or 1:1.6. Trust me when I say that, mathematically speaking, both of these are the same thing.

So I want my central incisor to have a length to width ratio of 1 to 0.6, where 1 is the height and 0.6 is the width. The central incisor is also a bigger tooth then the one next to it (the lateral incisor);

and the widths of the teeth relative to each other should also be in golden proportion, with the width of the central incisor being 1 and the width of the lateral incisor 0.6.

I will often see patients who have very worn down teeth who tell me that that their smile does not look nice any more, despite their teeth still looking straight and white. What has happened is that because the teeth are worn down, the proportions do not look right any more. The wear on the edge of the tooth causes the front teeth to either look square, or with very severe wear, they can even look rectangular but with their width being longer than their height. These smiles do not look right at all.

Fixing these smiles can sometimes take a large amount of treatment because you often find that the tooth wear is the same at the back of the mouth as it is at the front. Sometimes these patients need to have restorations on all of their teeth in order to give them back the smile and the function they once had.

Position of the smile in the face

It is important to assess if the smile is too high or too low, or too far out or too far in the mouth. This is best done by taking photos from specific angles and also by taking some videos of the patient speaking so that you can get an idea of the way that the smile looks in motion.

Then a simple diagnosis is made with a treatment plan. One example is when the position of the teeth is too low so too much gum shows when somebody is smiling. This 'gummy' smile can look quite unattractive and needs specific treatment called crown lengthening to improve the appearance. If this treatment is not done before restorations are placed, the treatment will not look very good even when it is completed. Likewise, if the smile is too high and you cannot see any of the teeth when somebody is smiling fully, it is important to remember to make the teeth look longer so that they are visible. If the teeth are too far in the face, it can give a sunken appearance and look like the lip has no support. In this case we may need to do orthodontics (braces) to move the teeth or provide slightly thicker restorations so that we can give more fullness to the lip. If the teeth protrude too much, the patient will have a 'goofy' appearance.

Again, this must be recognised before planning treatment so that measures can be made to try and manage/alter the appearance as long as the patient is aware and wishes for this to be changed. It is important that these planned alterations are conveyed to a patient before the final restorations are made so that the patient is aware of what he/she is going to get before it's delivered.

Normally this is done by creating what we call 'provisional' teeth. The patient is able to wear these for some time so as to ascertain whether he/she is happy with the smile before the final restorations are made.

Crowded teeth

Crowding happens when the teeth that are present, take up more space than there is available in the mouth. The upper and lower teeth are arranged in roughly a horseshoe shape called the dental arch. If, for example, the arch width is 10 cm and you have 11 teeth each at 1 cm long, they are not all going to fit into the arch. This is often the case and so the body compensates; rotating some of the teeth around or by having some of the teeth a little bit further forward or little bit further back. The teeth muddle together and just fit in!

The problem is these rotated and mal-aligned crowded teeth do not look very attractive. This is the most common reason why people come and see me when they are unhappy with their smile.

This issue is normally relatively straightforward to fix and we have two main ways of doing it. One is by providing orthodontic (braces) treatment. Braces work by putting forces on the teeth so that we move the teeth into better positions so they look more aligned. Normally we polish a little bit in between all of the teeth so that each of the teeth is a little bit narrower. This helps them to fit in very nicely into that arch we were talking about earlier.

This treatment works very nicely if the teeth are of good proportion and good colour (although whitening is often done after the braces have finished). Orthodontic treatment is an excellent way of managing crowded teeth because it is very simple to do and does not involve much destruction of the tooth. Braces can be done in a variety of different ways. You can have removable braces, clear aligners or metal, or tooth-coloured fixed braces. Some systems can be quite slow in moving the teeth and others can be much quicker.

My advice would always be to use a brace system that moves the crown and the root of the tooth properly, not just the crown of the tooth (the biting part). The end point of treatment should be when the root of the tooth is properly aligned, as well as the crown. When the root of the tooth is aligned it means that the result is far more stable because the root will be at the correct angle and held securely within the bone. Although not always guaranteed, it is much less likely for the teeth to relapse when the root position is correct.

I use a system which aligns the whole tooth, so the crown and the root are positioned in the correct place in the bone. Because this movement happens very efficiently, the treatment is much quicker than with conventional braces. With this system, the job is done properly and in a fraction of the time; in months rather than years.

The problem was that for a long time, we as dentists thought that if more force was put onto the teeth, they would move more quickly. Actually, the opposite is true. When light forces are applied to the teeth, they seem to move much more rapidly through the bone. The braces I use work quickly because they have managed to control the amount of force placed on each tooth so that it is not overloaded. This also has the benefit of considerably less pain when the teeth are moving.

Braces, generally, do have some disadvantages. Obviously, the fixed braces cannot be removed and that means that the appearance of the teeth can be compromised while the treatment is active. Although there is an option to have clear fixed braces, the truth is that they can also be seen, especially close up.

It is also hard to keep the teeth clean when wearing braces because there are more irregular surfaces and areas where plaque and food can be trapped. The final problem is that sometimes you can have situations where brackets can pop off, especially if patients eat hard food or grind their teeth. (More on tooth grinding and clenching in Chapter 11.) This can lead to more visits than planned at the outset of treatment.

Overall, though, braces are great and I love providing this kind of treatment because the change from how a smile was before treatment compared to how it is at the end can sometimes be overwhelming. It is so nice to be able to do treatment that genuinely makes patients really happy and yields such a noticeable result.

FREE BONUS

Visit the book website www.smilingdentist.co.uk to link to my practice for a free orthodontic consultation with me or one of my highly trained dentists.
(Remember to bring your book with you so that it can be signed.)

The alternative to having braces to align crooked teeth is to place veneers on them. If the crowded teeth are very skilfully smoothed down and restorations are placed on them, it can give the illusion of having a lovely straight smile. The only disadvantage is that as we mentioned earlier, it can be destructive.

If, for example, the crowding means that one of the teeth has really ended up having to stick out a long way, then we may have to smooth a considerable amount of that tooth down before we can make it look straight and part of an attractive smile. This can have consequences for the tooth like the nerve in the tooth dying. In extreme cases, it could even potentially lead to the loss of the tooth.

However, if after the teeth are straightened, their proportions still look poor, then veneers do offer the advantage of managing the size and shape as well as the colour and also giving the appearance of straight teeth. In these cases, veneers or crowns are definitely the treatment of choice. Sometimes, the best choice is a combination treatment of braces followed by veneers or crowns. This has the overwhelming advantage that by moving the teeth first, we can minimise the tooth reduction because the teeth will virtually be in the correct positions before the veneer treatment starts.

When designing a smile and doing smile makeover treatment, it is of course, important for the dentist to have sound knowledge of what makes a smile look nice. But I think it is more important for the dentist to really communicate well with the patient so that he/she is able to precisely know what you as the patient wants so that you are happy with the final outcome. Whether it be a verbal explanation or the use of visual aids, or the trial smile that we mentioned earlier we should always know where we are heading before we get there.

Veneers are a great treatment which can be prescribed to treat many of the deficient smile situations outlined above. Fantastic results can be achieved when tooth proportions are incorrect like worn teeth or where adjacent teeth are different sizes, or if there are symmetry issues. Veneers can also be used to correct crowded and rotated teeth and also when a colour match is wrong. Placement of veneers normally does involve some tooth smoothing but a very pleasing result can be obtained. And it is considerably quicker than having orthodontic treatments.

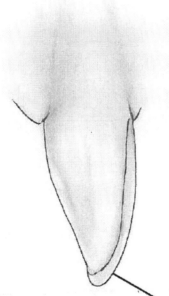

Amount of Tooth Smoothed Away to make space for Veneer

ILLUSTRATION OF THE SIDE OF AN INCISOR TOOTH SHOWING A VENEER ON THE FRONT OF THE TOOTH.
NOTE HOW THIN THE VENEER IS AND HOW LITTLE TOOTH NEEDS TO BE SMOOTHED AWAY IN ORDER TO PROVIDE IT

When doing veneer treatment, it is often helpful to have an idea of how we want the smile to be before we start doing any tooth reduction so that both the dentist and patient can be sure that the result they are going to get is something everyone will be happy with before any tooth smoothing has been done. Once a clear decision has been made, the procedure involves polishing away a very small amount of the tooth substance. An impression is taken so that a model can be made and sent to the lab where the veneers are individually fabricated.

Veneers are made out of porcelain which is a great tooth replacement material because it so closely resembles the tooth structure. The material can be made in a variety of colours to match the teeth but it has a crystalline structure similar to tooth enamel. This means that the way it interacts with light, i.e. refraction and reflection of different wavelengths of light, is the same as the interaction between enamel and light. This property allows veneers to look just like teeth if they are skilfully provided.

Temporary veneers can be placed onto the teeth so that patients have a nice smile in between the two appointments. The second appointment is normally made one-two weeks after the first appointment. This is when the final veneers can be bonded in place.

Veneers and orthodontic treatment are normally the two most appropriate options for patients with healthy teeth. Sometimes the teeth can be infected, painfull, or wobbly and cannot be saved; yet it is the poor appearance of these hopeless teeth, rather than the functional problems, that motivates the patient to attend. Options for this type of treatment may be more drastic and involve the removal of some teeth, but this will be covered in more detail in the next chapter.

Chapter 7

"I Have Missing Teeth. Can I Replace Them?"

I can show you what options you have and how you can smile and bite with confidence again.

Do we Always Need to Replace Teeth?

Many people are either missing teeth in their mouths or they may present to the dentist requiring removal of a tooth/teeth.

We as dentists are aware that not only is this a traumatic experience, but it can also be quite psychologically damaging: one with connotations of getting older and the stigma attached to not having all of your teeth, especially if a front tooth is lost. The good news is there are some very good replacements for teeth which can not only restore the mouth but also the lost confidence.

When I speak to patients, I always outline four separate options for replacing teeth that have been lost:

1. Leave a gap
2. Make a denture
3. Place a bridge
4. Place a dental implant

In some instances, leaving a gap is the best option. There are times when removal of a tooth, especially at the back of the mouth, will not cause any functional problems. The patient will find that, even without that tooth, they are still able to eat and chew anything that they were able to eat before. In these circumstances, we often advise the patient to leave the gap, as long as he/she is aware that sometimes the teeth next to the gap, or the tooth opposing the gap can move. Sometimes this can have consequences for the bite and the way that the mouth is able to move.

In fact, there is a concept called the 'shortened dental arch' which advises that in some instances it is possible for patients to eat a completely full and varied diet without having the back teeth. So you do not always have to feel pressured that if a tooth comes out, that a replacement is always needed.

Types of Replacement

A **denture** is a type of false tooth which is normally made out of plastic or metal. It is a plate that rests either on the gum or on the other teeth.

Dentures have the advantage that they are relatively cheap to construct and they can be used to restore many teeth at the same time. However, dentures do not have any fixed anchor points so they do not function like teeth, and hence must be regarded as something of a compromise. Unlike natural teeth which have roots which anchor into the bone, a denture is a plate that sits on the surface of the gum so it will normally not feel as secure as biting with either fixed teeth or fixed replacement teeth (this will be covered later in this chapter).

Dentures can be bulky and encroach upon the space where the tongue normally likes to be. Also, there are many taste buds on the roof of the mouth and as the top denture normally covers the roof of the mouth, it can make it hard for patients to taste their food.

Food can get trapped underneath the dentures, and hence after eating a meal it may be necessary to take the dentures out so that they can be cleaned. They can rub and be sore. Sometimes it is necessary to use some kind of 'fixative' or denture adhesive in order to keep the dentures in place securely. Dentures do need to be removed so that they can be cleaned and often patients will remove them at night for comfort. This also gives an opportunity for oxygen to get to the skin underneath the denture.

Some of the above objections can be overcome by constructing a metal denture. Metal dentures are much stronger and can be very thin with a minimal framework. This helps to prevent the denture from encroaching upon the space within the mouth reducing that feeling of bulkiness. A window can often be cut in the plate so that the roof of the mouth is exposed allowing the patient to taste food. Clips and clasps are normally incorporated into the framework design and these can be used to help the denture positively click on to some of the teeth so that the denture feels more secure and does not rock and slide around as much when it's being used. Patients who have been using plastic dentures will often change to metal dentures and are normally very happy with the new denture because of the improvements it makes to their quality of life.

Another option is a **bridge**. A bridge is a fixed tooth replacement which uses existing healthy teeth to help to hold on the new false teeth.

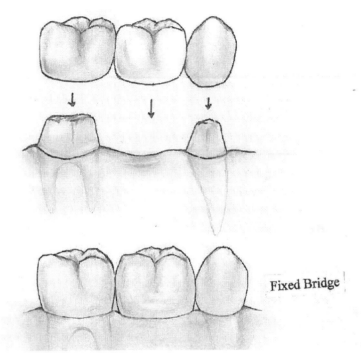

ILLUSTRATION OF A BRIDGE SHOWING HOW THE TEETH EITHER SIDE
OF THE GAP CAN BE SMOOTHED DOWN SO THAT THEY CAN HELP TO
RETAIN A FALSE TOOTH

A bridge can be a great option because it does not need a plate; does not cover the roof of the mouth at all or encroach upon the tongue space. Because they are fixed, bridges do not need to be removed to be cleaned. They are brushed and flossed in a very similar way to natural teeth. Bridges can be used to restore gaps of all sizes, from one missing tooth, all the way up to very large gaps of many missing teeth.

Bridges can be retained by having a small wing which is glued onto the teeth next to the gap. Or the teeth which are holding the bridge can be smoothed down like they are when crowns are made, and the crowns can be used to hold the bridge on. This means they will have a much more positive grip but potentially do involve more removal of the tooth structure.

Both options have their advantages and disadvantages. Often when I assess the situation one will have a particular overriding advantage so this kind of judgement is normally made on a case-by-case basis.

Bridges can be very nice looking restorations. Often if a patient has a number of mal-aligned or crooked front teeth which are very bad, those teeth can be removed and replaced with a bridge with nice, straight teeth. Like most restorations, the colour of the bridge is normally matched to the existing teeth to look seamless within the smile.

Dental implants are the type of replacement for missing teeth which most mimic a natural tooth. The implant is made up of a screw that is held within the jaw bone (this mimics the root of the tooth and acts as an anchor for the artificial tooth) and the artificial crown which is held onto the buried implant screw. This artificial crown is designed to function like a tooth and also mimics the way a tooth looks. It is a great restoration that looks very realistic, but also the implant is anchored in place onto the implant screw so it bites and functions like a real tooth, too.

The advantages of dental implants are that they tend to be very long lasting restorations and provide the most life-like replacement for missing teeth. The treatment does not require cutting down any of the healthy teeth next to the gap. The implant helps to preserve the mass of the jawbone, so it does not shrink away giving that 'sunken-in' look that some people can have after losing teeth.

When fully discussing implant treatment, patients often have the same reservations so I would like to highlight these now. Dental implant treatment does involve some dental surgery because the first step in the treatment is to place the implant screw into the bone. Another factor to remember is that dental implant treatment can be costly. As long as these two objections can be overcome, and the treatment is suitable, it can begin.

Regarding suitability, a full assessment of the mouth must be done before thinking about placing implants because there are some patients where implants can be prone to failure. For example, with smokers or people with long standing gum disease, the success rate for implant treatment is lower. But it is important to take a view of the whole mouth even if placing a single implant into a single space.

Implants are very versatile. They can be used to retain bridges. So if the teeth are poor candidates for holding on a bridge, two implants can be placed and used to hold on many more teeth.

Implants can also be used to help to support or retain dentures. Lower dentures can be very difficult restorations for patients to get on with. If the bone has shrunk away so that the denture has only a flat surface to hold onto, the tongue and the lips can move the lower denture very easily and create a very difficult set of teeth to bite on. Implants can be placed under the denture and used to anchor it in place. This is a great treatment, and again, is one that can really improve a patient's quality of life.

Implant

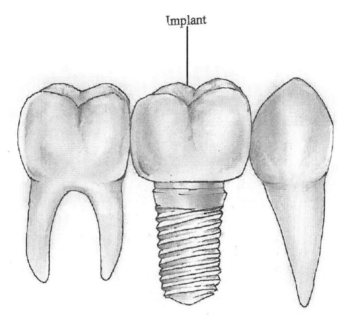

ILLUSTRATION OF A DENTAL IMPLANT-SUPPORTED-CROWN SHOWING THE DENTAL IMPLANT, WHICH MIMICS THE ROOT OF A NATURAL TOOTH, AND THE CROWN, WHICH LOOKS VERY SIMILAR TO AND FUNCTIONS AS A NATURAL TOOTH CROWN DOES

Chapter 8

"I Have Painful Wisdom Teeth. What Should I Do?"

I will go through the treatment options and discuss when it is best to remove a wisdom tooth.

Painful wisdom teeth are one of the most common problems I see. The reason they are so common is because of evolution. As time has gone on, we have evolved a much softer diet than our ancestors and, as such, our jaws have started to shrink. This means that, whereas once upon a time, the wisdom teeth would fit very nicely into the jaws, now more often than not, our smaller jaws do not allow enough space for the wisdom teeth to fully come through. Problems normally arise because the wisdom teeth are half in and half out; and we would classify these teeth as 'partially erupted'.

When the wisdom tooth is half out, it is often covered by flap of gum and it can be very easy for food and plaque to stagnate around that gum and the wisdom tooth can become infected. When this happens, it can be very sore, and certainly much more painful than the discomfort you get when a wisdom tooth is simply coming through (erupting). This kind of pain can be helped by rinsing with warm salty water, but often it does need some medicine to resolve it.

It would be advisable to see a dentist, if this kind of problem arises, to assess the situation, ensure it is this type of infection and prescribe the medicine that is correct for you.

If this becomes a recurrent problem, there is an option of removing the wisdom teeth. There are instances where swelling and infection associated with the gum surrounding the lower wisdom tooth can be made worse if a top wisdom tooth is then able to bite upon the swollen gum. When this happens, often a choice needs to be made as to which tooth (upper or lower) needs to be removed. Given the choice between removal of the top wisdom tooth and bottom wisdom tooth, I will often make the decision to remove the top wisdom tooth. This is because the top wisdom tooth is normally one of the easier teeth to remove, and hence there is very little pain, swelling, or bruising after having the treatment done. Lower wisdom teeth are often more difficult to remove.

When people mention having the wisdom teeth out and how difficult it was, they are normally referring to the lower wisdom teeth.

Partially erupted wisdom teeth can also be very difficult to clean and can cause food traps which can affect other teeth, notably the molar teeth in front of the wisdom teeth. This food trapping can sometimes lead to decay in both of these molar teeth. If this kind of thing is happening, then that would also be a very good reason to have the lower wisdom teeth removed.

Removal of a lower wisdom tooth is a more involved procedure with its difficulty being affected by the orientation of the tooth and how far out the tooth is. Another factor influencing difficulty is whether there is any bone or gum in the way of the tooth.

There is also an important nerve called the Inferior Dental (I.D.) nerve which can be very close to the root of the lower wisdom tooth. That is why it is mandatory to take an x-ray of the tooth before deciding to remove it. This helps to ensure that it is not too close to that nerve and thus risk damaging the nerve during the procedure. However, it is important to appreciate that there is always a very small risk that there may be some nerve damage when carrying out this procedure.

Chapter 9

"I Have Something on My Gum. Is It Oral Cancer?"

I can explain what oral cancer looks like, what to be concerned about, and what you should get checked out.

Thankfully oral cancer is very rare, but it is very serious.

If allowed to spread oral cancer is often fatal. But if caught early, survival rates are very good. I feel that for this reason alone, regular attendance at the dentist is something that is really important, so that routine screening of the oral soft tissues can be performed by a dentist.

The skin in the mouth (the 'Oral Mucosa') is very similar to the skin elsewhere in the body. As such, there are many things that can appear on the skin in the mouth like ulcers, bumps, and lumps along with white and red patches. Most of these are completely harmless and often disappear as quickly as they appear.

There are certain things that appear in the mouth that a dentist might be particularly worried about, but if we rely on visual inspection it can be impossible to be completely sure.

Dentists, however, are particularly cautious and if we feel even a little bit troubled by what we see, we will normally refer the patient to a specialist for a second opinion. If the specialist is also concerned, then they can perform what is called a 'biopsy'. This is a procedure where a small part of the affected skin is removed and sent to a laboratory where special tests are performed, then the tissue is observed under a microscope. Here, the appearance can be scrutinised and the specialist can see what is happening at a cellular level. It gives assurance to see if everything is okay or if, indeed, there is a problem.

When dentists examine a patient's mouth, there are certain things that we look for that may worry us. (This is by no means a categorical or exhaustive list, but I hope it gives some idea of the things we may choose to refer to a specialist.) These things include something like a lump or bump that is growing very rapidly; an ulcer that stays for more than 3 weeks (especially if the ulcer is not painful); and a lesion with a very disordered appearance, (i.e. it is made up of many different colours).

There are certain things that can increase a patient's risk of getting oral cancer and the most common is smoking. The chemicals within the smoke will affect the skin in the mouth and irritate it. It is this irritation that can cause the changes which lead to cancer. Drinking alcohol, especially spirits, is also linked with causing oral cancer. The theory is that the spirit has the effect of thinning the skin in the mouth. Irritants that would not normally penetrate the skin are able to penetrate the now thinned and permeable skin.

The biggest risk factor is smoking and drinking alcohol together. These two actions have what we call a 'synergistic' effect which means that they are much more than simply the sum of their parts. They end up having a multiplier effect. Other habits like chewing tobacco and 'Paan' (Betel quid) are also well linked with an increase in oral cancer.

I would always advise patients that if they are at all worried about anything in their mouths, then it is best and safest to get it checked out. Most of the time, the patients are told that everything is fine. But as mentioned, time plays such a large part in whether the cancer is curable or not, that it pays to get things looked at sooner rather than later.

Chapter 10

"I'm Nervous, Will It Hurt?"

I will go through how I treat nervous patients and how I am able to perform virtually painless dentistry.

Modern dentistry has come a very long way.

I have many patients who have seen the dentist either as children or have not been to see the dentist for a long time. These patients often talk about specific bad experiences that they had and how this has 'put them off' from seeing the dentist until now.

First, I would like to explain that I do enjoy treating nervous patients. I love being able to put somebody at ease and slowly (or quickly) watch their confidence grow through doing small treatments and potentially building up to things that are little bit more complicated.

When patients are nervous, I will always ask exactly what it is about being at the dentist that they do not like. I do this because I think that in these situations, to overcome these difficult interactions, clarity is everything.

If there was a specific problem that a previous dentist caused, then I want to be absolutely sure not to make the same mistake again. I feel that by explaining this to the patient from the outset, it serves to give the patient some confidence that I am sensitive to their situation and will do all that I can to help them and work with them.

I have the greatest respect for patients who are nervous and still attend. I once heard a quote that . . . *"courage is not the absence of fear, it is feeling fearful yet taking action anyway"*.

That is exactly what these patients are doing and I commend them for it and will work with them as well as I can.

Broadly speaking, patients fall into one of the three categories: Those who are nervous about injections, those who are nervous about drilling and the potential pain that it can cause, and those who are nervous about the loss of control when somebody is working in their mouths. Each of these difficulties can be managed. Let me explain how I try to help patients overcome their difficulties.

Fear develops into a 'phobia' when one feels that they lack the resource to overcome a particular challenge. When we feel unable to face something, then the only alternative is avoidance. Some of my patients have been avoiding the dentist for far too long, so when they finally do present, they come with really bad problems, and often pain. This constant pain is the only motivation that overcomes their desire to avoid that difficult, almost impossible situation.

Once a patient in this level of difficulty has sought my help, I feel it is my duty to help them to overcome any difficulties. I show the patient that he/she does have the tools within them to meet any challenge whilst in the dental chair. If this is done well, one can turn highly phobic patients into patients who attend regularly and are either ambivalent about, or indeed enjoy, attending.

If patients are nervous about injections, there are a number of ways we can try to get around it. When doing particularly small fillings or small treatments, we may elect to avoid injecting altogether. Another simple way of helping is to try to ensure that the patient keeps his/her eyes closed, because often it is the site of the needle which sparks all the fears. Use of topical anaesthetic gel can also help because it will numb the gum superficially before the needle goes in, and this can make the experience much more comfortable.

The major reason why injections are painful is not the needle piercing the skin, however, it is actually the pressure build-up when the local anaesthetic solution is introduced into the tissues. That is why I routinely inject very, very slowly so that I can reduce this pressure build-up until it is almost negligible.

Another great technique is to try and distract the tissues away from the sensation of the needle piercing the skin. There are different types of nerve fibres which conduct pain signals to the brain. There are 'A' fibres and 'C' fibres. 'A' fibres are quicker fibres and they will conduct sensation in preference to the 'C' fibre. The 'C' fibres are normally responsible for conducting the sensation of pain from injections to the brain. 'A' fibres will also conduct this pain but also tell the brain about the sensation of touch. When dentists are aware of this then they can sometimes strategically pinch or wiggle the lip. This means that the brain becomes preoccupied with feeling the pinch or the movement and so forgets about the pain of the injection.

If these techniques are used correctly, I am very happy to say, that many patients will ask 'have you started yet?' **after** I have finished injecting. That is one of the most satisfying parts of my job, i.e. when I know that the patient has not felt anything so the injection has not hurt at all.

One area I do find difficult to numb, without any pain, is the upper front teeth. The tissues are very tight here and so even the introduction of a drop of local anaesthetic is normally felt. I really try to coach patients and explain that there will be some discomfort when numbing this area, as the last thing I ever want to do is to lie to a patient and promise that something is going to be painless when it will not be. I feel this is the quickest way to lose someone's trust.

The technique I use at the front of the mouth is to introduce a very small drop of anaesthetic into the gum and then stop and wait between 20 or 30 seconds. I find that, in this time, the gum normally goes very numb, and then I am able to reintroduce the needle once again and it does not cause any pain the second time. Therefore, I am able to introduce the rest of the anaesthetic (enough so that the tooth will go numb) painlessly. While on the topic of numbing, I will often have a talk with patients about what they will feel when their mouth is numbed, especially if it is the first time that they have ever experienced this.

Local anaesthetic solution works by blocking the signals that the nerve fibres convey to the brain telling the brain about touch and pain. There are other nerve fibres called motor neurones which are responsible for moving muscles. In dentistry, we are most concerned with blocking the nerves that convey pain and sensation. When this is done successfully, you find that for the first 30 seconds to 2 minutes after the injection, there will be a feeling of pins and needles. After that, it develops into the feeling of 'fatness' or numbness (as if the part that has been numbed has swollen). Although it may feel like the lip is extremely big, I will often show the patient how they look in the mirror so that they can see that the anaesthetic has no effect on the way things look, only on the way things feel.

Another thing I will explain to patients is how the bone in the upper jaw and in the lower jaw is very different. In the upper jaw the bone is very porous, almost like sponge. This means that if we inject local anaesthetic right next to the tooth, it will be soaked up through the bone and gets right next to the root of the tooth. Therefore, it numbs the tooth effectively.

However, in the lower jaw, the bone is much denser (almost like granite) so if we deposit local anaesthetic next to the tooth, we find that it does not always numb the tooth effectively.

For teeth in the lower jaw, we often adopt a slightly different technique, whereby we numb the nerve that supplies all of the teeth in the lower jaw on one side. This is called a 'block injection'.

Not only do the teeth go numb, but also the lower lip and the tongue (but only on the side that has been numbed). So numbing for the lower teeth feels far more extensive than it does for the upper teeth. It is important for patients to be aware of this difference before they start, so that they know that it is normal, and everything is okay.

Another important point to make is that if we need to do some treatment on a lower tooth on the right-hand side, and then also a lower tooth on the left-hand side, then we need to make at least two separate appointments to do these treatments so that we do not numb the whole of the lower jaw in one go. It is very unpleasant for patients to have the whole lower jaw numb because they would not be able to feel their lip or tongue at all and could even end up biting or chewing their lip or tongue.

I think that if a dentist can learn to numb patients effectively, and as close to painlessly as possible, then they can treat their patients very well, especially nervous patients. It is so fundamental to delivering good dentistry and underpins all treatment. If patients are numbed properly, they will have so much confidence in their dentist and the treatment they provide. This will go a long way in helping them to become confident and regular attenders.

If the problem is drilling or pain, you often find there is a history of previous dental work where a dentist has drilled the patient's tooth, and it has caused pain while the treatment was carried out. When this happens, the brain often links the pain of the drill with the sound and the vibration of the drill. This can create what psychologists call an 'anchor'. Often patients can be in the waiting area and when they hear that high-pitched sound of the drill, they will experience a 'state change' and feel very anxious. It is as if the sound makes them feel the pain they felt when the anchor was made.

When this has happened in the past, it is important to introduce a new anchor; one where confidence and comfort are linked to the sound of drill. This is done with effective numbing and by stopping work when patients feel pain.

This is often very closely linked to those patients who feel like they lose control. They often feel that if the procedure is painful, the dentist will continue even if they request the dentist to stop. Or they feel like they may not be able to communicate to the dentist that they want it stopped right now.

In my experience, I find that a slow and explanatory approach can be very helpful along with giving a 'safe signal'. I inform my patients that if they raise their hand while I am working, then I will stop, no matter what. Patients can request to stop to have a breather, if their mouth is filling with water or indeed if they are feeling any pain or sensitivity.

Often, I encourage patients to test me and to just raise their hand whenever they feel like it, just to be sure that I really will stop. When I do (and I always do), I really find that patients start to learn to trust once again.

I feel really proud if I am able to turn a nervous patient into a patient who is able to attend and have routine dentistry done, without any help other than local anaesthetic and a bit of tender loving care. There are, of course, patients who will still not be able to have dentistry done under those circumstances. There are a number of techniques that can be used to help for these patients.

Patients can be given nitrous oxide (laughing gas) which helps to relax them when they are having dentistry done, or they can have sedation which is a special medicine either taken orally or injected into a vein. I often joke with patients that having sedation is a little bit like downing two bottles of red wine! When a patient has sedation, they have very little awareness of what is happening, but they also have an amnesic effect, as well. So they, happily, have very little recollection of the procedure.

Sedation is very handy not only for nervous patients having routine dentistry but also for confident patients who, perhaps, have to have a particularly difficult procedure done. (Possibly, it is used for surgery or for very long dental treatments.) There is also the option of having a general anaesthetic for dental treatment, but this has become far more uncommon now and would have to be provided in a hospital and not in a general dental practice.

It is also becoming more common for dentists to be trained in hypnosis. Many of the techniques taught in hypnosis can really help very nervous dental patients to relax. Hypnosis can also help patients gain the ability to cope when a patient feels that they do not have that ability.

I do hope that by reading this chapter, some patients who may have feared coming to the dentist may decide that they are now able to. Hopefully, as a patient you will understand that some dentists do have a really good understanding of what can make people nervous and they will do their best to really try and help patients. They want patients to attend and to have any and all required treatment done.

Chapter 11

"Am I Grinding My Teeth?"

I will show you what to look out for, to find out if this destructive habit is affecting your teeth.

Tooth grinding and clenching known as 'Bruxism' or 'Parafunction' is a very common problem, but one that very few patients know is happening. It can be incredibly destructive leading to a variety of serious problems.

Only very few patients are aware of it because it tends to happen in the middle of the night in the deepest part of the sleep cycle. This makes it difficult for the patient to recall actually grinding or clenching. Apart from the dentist, often it is the patient's spouse or partner who knows first when the patient is grinding or clenching. Perhaps the patient will wake up with certain signs or symptoms but be unaware that it is caused by bruxing.

When patients clench or grind, tremendous force is put into what we call the 'Masticatory system'. This is how we describe the machine that is our mouth.

People will often be predisposed to having a weak point in that system. The system includes the teeth, the gums, the jaw joints, and the muscles that move the jaw.

If, for instance, the patient has gum disease, one might find that the gums show the sign of weakness, and eventually the teeth end up wobbling. Sometimes the teeth are heavily filled or weak and so they end up either wearing down, or they can start breaking down and bits can break off. If the muscles are affected, patients can often wake up with headaches which can be quite severe. Patients can think these headaches are caused by other diseases or problems.

If the jaw joints are affected, sometimes they can exhibit a sign that we call 'Crepitus' which is like a creaking or cracking as the patient is opening or closing the mouth. Sometimes patients might find that they are unable to open their mouth as wide as they used to be able to. Some patients find that they are unable to chew particularly chewy foods like gum, bagels, or steak and that the jaw becomes very tired and painful if they do. This can also affect patient's ability to keep their mouths open especially when they are having dental treatment done.

I would like to qualify at this point that clicking jaws is very common and not always attributed to tooth grinding or clenching.

There is a lot of controversy surrounding tooth grinding because it is very difficult to find a consensus opinion amongst dentists as to what causes it. This means that dentists disagree about what actually causes it!

There are some that believe it is caused wholly by an incorrect bite. Others believe that is caused completely by stress.

However, the majority of dentists do agree that there is some component in the way we bite and some component in stress which causes this.

When we, as dentists, talk about 'Occlusion' or the bite, we are talking about the relationship between the upper jaw which is fused to the skull (and hence does not move) and the lower jaw which can move.

When we bite up and down with the jaw joints in the correct position, (dentists call this 'centric relation' or 'habit bite'), the upper and lower teeth do not necessarily contact evenly. It is more common that as your jaws close, there would be only one contact between your teeth, and this would normally be between one of your top and bottom back teeth.

Therefore, the lower jaw changes its position, ever so slightly, so that all the teeth can meet and share the load of the bite evenly. If it did not, there would be too much force going through the teeth where there is that one contact and it would be very painful. When the jaw manipulates itself into this new position of the best bite, however, it can pull one or both of the jaw joints out of position slightly. When this happens, it is not painful immediately, but it sets up stress in the joint and in the muscles.

This stress may not be enough to cause grinding or clenching on its own, but if added to other stress like external stress from work or from life, in general, it can cause us to go over a threshold level and then the bruxing can start.

This threshold level can be different for different people, and hence some people are more prone to bruxing then others.

Indeed, if the patient has a very low threshold level but very large discrepancy in where their jaw joint position is, this may be enough for them to start grinding without needing any external stress at all. On the other hand, some people may have a threshold level that is so high that they never grind or clench their teeth.

If dentists can determine that patients are clenching and grinding their teeth, then one sensible way to treat them is to try and correct this discrepancy in the bite. The simplest way this can be done is to provide a guard or an appliance that patients would normally wear at night-time. The way it works is that it fits securely over the teeth. (I normally make them to fit over the lower teeth but guards can also be made to fit over the upper teeth, too.) It is designed in such a way, that when the jaw joints are in their correct positions, the upper teeth meet against and guard evenly. This means that when the patient wears the guard, the most comfortable place for them to bite will also be where the jaw joints are in the correct position and the muscles are relaxed. By removing this stress on the system, the impetus to want to clench or grind is removed.

This treatment works particularly well with patients presenting with tension headaches caused by the muscles involved in tooth grinding. Often we find that the headaches disappear altogether, and very quickly, after making this type of guard.

The beauty of the treatment is that if the bruxing stops, then all of the destructive aspects associated with the bruxing will stop, too. Often patients ask me if the appliance is too uncomfortable to wear at night, but my experience has been that when patients stop grinding they often find that they sleep better and that any pain they had previously resolves. Eventually, they often find that they are unable to sleep without the guard.

Chapter 12

"Are My Children's Teeth Alright?"

How to assess if children's teeth are okay
and what do I do if a tooth is knocked out?

Children's dentistry

It is really important for parents to bring children to see the dentist regularly for a number of reasons. Of course, it is important for dentists to examine children's mouths, so that we can make sure that all is well with regard to dental health and also tooth development. But it is also really important for children to come regularly so that it develops a good habit of seeing the dentist at regular intervals for routine examinations. This allows us to give preventative advice but also means that if problems are detected, they are done so in a timely fashion so that less invasive treatments can be done when problems are still small.

When parents attend with children, I am often asked the same questions about the timing of teeth erupting, about whether teeth are crowded, and whether the children will need braces or not. These are great questions and I understand completely why parents are concerned and want to know that all is developing well. In this chapter, I will attempt to briefly outline the advice I give to patients but hope that it will not be used as a substitute to taking your children to see the dentist.

We normally expect the first set of teeth to come out between six months and three years of age. Generally it is the lower front teeth that come out first followed by the upper front teeth. More teeth will erupt going backwards in the mouth until eventually, between two and three years of age, the child's last molar tooth comes through.

Generally speaking, the mechanics of the teething process is normally very straightforward. However, because of the age of the child, it can be a very trying time for the child and also for the parents because it is always associated with pain and difficulty with eating. It can also be associated with high-temperature diarrhoea, ear pain, and a generally very tough time for all involved.

On average, adult teeth come through at around six years of age and you expect the lower front teeth to be the first ones to appear.

The point should be made that, we as dentists are taught at dental school, the range of ages that we expect certain teeth to erupt. As I became more experienced, however, I realised that these age ranges do not always apply and that often I was worrying patients unduly, based upon the knowledge I had gained. I would be explaining that teeth were erupting late, but then they would erupt (often only after a few more months).

I soon learned that the timing of eruption is far less important than the order in which the teeth come out. If the order is incorrect, especially with the very front and back teeth, that can often be something that is worth investigating because it can mean that those teeth are not present or that something is stopping them from coming through. That is often why the next tooth in the sequence has come out before the missing one.

Normally, when this happens, the dentist would take an x-ray to see what is going on 'behind the scenes'. This would help to ascertain if the teeth are present or impeded in any way within the bone. The x-ray allows us to plan any intervention if it is needed.

After the lower front teeth (central incisors) come through, you normally expect the upper central incisors to erupt. After that, you would expect the teeth next to the lower front teeth (the lateral incisors) to come through, and then you expect the upper lateral incisors to follow.

Whilst this is all happening at the front, the jaw also grows quite significantly. This makes space at the back of the mouth for the first adult molar teeth to come through. No teeth are lost in order for these teeth to come through; and so it is a little bit less dramatic than at the front where the baby teeth are lost before the adult teeth come through. However, children of this age will often complain of discomfort at the back of the mouth, or perhaps even an earache, as these back teeth come through.

After the adult incisors and the adult molar teeth have come through, things go 'quiet' for a couple of years and we do not lose any more teeth. Normally, at around age nine (remember this number is only there to give a very rough guide), we start losing the first set of baby back teeth and baby canines. These are replaced by the adult canines and the adult premolar teeth. It is at around this age that we are able to plan whether a patient will need braces or not. The reason we wait until this time is that before this point, normally we can only guess. This is because we do not know how big the teeth will be that come through or how much the jaws will grow.

Children may need braces for a variety of reasons. If it is because of a mismatch in the jaw sizes, i.e. if the lower jaw or the upper jaw is too big relative to the opposing jaw, then it is relatively easy to diagnose and plan that braces will be needed from a much earlier age. However, the most common reason for requiring braces when the jaws are of correct size is having the teeth within them either take up too much space or too little space. We call this 'crowding' or 'spacing' as touched on this in Chapter 6. Until all the adult teeth are through, we are unable to predict how big they will be. We are also unable to predict how much the jaws will grow and be able to accommodate these bigger teeth.

More often than not, patients will have very crowded-looking mouths up to a certain age, but frequently, after the jaws grow, the teeth are normally accommodated very well and straighten up beautifully without the need for braces.

Baby teeth, just like adult teeth, are made up of the crown of the tooth which is the bit that we can see and also a root which is buried in the jaw bone. When the adult tooth starts to grow, its journey is such that it will grow up through the gum where the root of the baby tooth was. When this happens, the root of the baby tooth shrinks away. We call this process 'resorption'.

As this resorption continues and the tooth root shrinks, the baby tooth becomes progressively less well held in, until eventually, it starts to wobble and then comes out. Soon after the baby tooth is lost, the adult tooth emerges from the gum and then continues to grow in to its correct position.

Sometimes as the adult tooth is growing up through the gum, it can grow up too close to the lip or too close to the tongue. When this happens, as it grows, it misses the baby tooth root, and hence, the trigger for the process of the baby root resorbing is not there. This means that there are situations when an adult tooth has appeared either behind or in front of a baby tooth and the baby tooth is still there, solidly positioned.

When this happens, the baby tooth can turn into a barrier which prevents the adult tooth from being positioned in the correct place. In this situation, it is often best for the baby tooth to be removed to allow the adult tooth to reposition. If the tooth removal is timed correctly, the adult tooth repositioning can happen spontaneously and avoid the need for braces.

Dental Trauma

I think it is very important for me to discuss first aid for teeth that have been traumatised. I find that this happens most commonly in children who have had trauma to the face, either from a fall or from a blow to the face. This can result in breaking or even completely losing a front tooth.

If a front tooth is broken, I would always encourage the patient to keep the broken bit. An appointment should be made with the dentist as soon as possible and the patient should bring the broken bit with them. From my point of view, it is always nice to see the bit of tooth. Sometimes, it can be glued back to the tooth and used as a temporary or permanent restoration (I have been surprised by how long some of these can last). Other times, it cannot be glued back, but it serves as a valuable guide for me to form the basis of the restoration that I make for the tooth.

When a tooth is knocked out, the initial management is very different depending on whether it is a baby tooth or an adult tooth. Remember, that the front adult teeth normally come through at around about six years old so this can be used as a guide. The reason I mention this is because it is not always the parents who are on hand to fix the problem. Commonly, it is a teacher or a football coach, and sometimes even a passer-by. That is why, if they can ascertain the age of the child affected, they can make an educated guess as to whether it is an adult tooth or a baby tooth.

If it is a baby tooth, you MUST NOT try to put the tooth back in again. Even the dentist would not do this. If a baby tooth has been knocked out, it must stay out. Any attempt to re-implant it can result in damage to the developing permanent tooth and that would be a disaster.

If, however, it is a permanent adult tooth that has come out, then the ideal treatment is to try and put it back into the socket as quickly as possible. It is important to try and clean the tooth first, but in doing so, do not scrub the tooth. Do not even handle the root of the tooth as this could damage the delicate cells which are needed to help the reattachment of the tooth back into the socket.

Early re-implantation is, by far, the best option and often leads to medium or long-term success. That means there is a good chance that the child will keep the tooth for a very long period of time.

If the tooth cannot be re-implanted at the site of the incident, then proper management of the tooth before seeing the dentist is critical. The best thing to do is to keep the tooth in the patient's mouth (tucked into the cheek is best). Saliva is the best preserver of those delicate cells on the root. The next best option is to put the tooth in some milk, if it is available, because milk will also help to preserve those cells.

Water is not the best option as it can often affect and damage those cells. Leaving the tooth out dry is the worst thing for it and will often result in the tooth being rejected even if it is put back in place.

Soon after the tooth is put back in, the nerve within the tooth will need to be removed and a root canal treatment performed.

The tooth will have to be reviewed many times and periodic x-rays taken to make sure that the tooth is not being rejected. If this rejection happens, a process called 'resorption' can happen and this can affect the root of the tooth or the bone surrounding it. This means that the root of the tooth or even the bone can shrink away. If this occurs the only viable treatment is to remove the tooth and to consider some type of replacement like a bridge or an implant.

Although an implant is normally the treatment of choice, this procedure would have to be delayed until the patient is fully grown because otherwise this can cause some complications.

That is why the initial appropriate management of the knocked out tooth is so important because if the re-implanted tooth can be kept for at least 10 years then we will have gotten to the age where the patient is fully grown. This means that we can start thinking about the type of options that will hopefully last a much longer amount of time (like a dental implant) if that re-implanted tooth fails.

FREE BONUS

Visit www.smilingdentist.co.uk to receive your free poster outlining what to do if someone you know knocks out or chips a tooth

I think that the general knowledge for what to do for a child if a front tooth is broken or knocked out is generally very poor. That is why I would like you to visit my website www.smilingdentist.co.uk and download a free poster which out-lines the immediate management of dental trauma when it occurs.

I would like a poster to be in every school, social club, chil-dren's football team, everywhere where children are and especially where they play. I would like all conscientious parents to give these posters to their local schools and clubs, so that if this trauma hap-pens to a child, there is a clear and easily understood poster to refer to. This will help people make the right decision and take the right action when some people may panic. I want this poster to become as commonplace as those great first-aid posters we see which help people to make the right decisions when other emergencies happen like management of cuts and bruises, or choking.

I hope that as a reader of my book, you will support this cause because although we will not save lives with these posters, it could potentially improve the quality of life for many children to whom this happens.

I also hope you have enjoyed reading my book and that you found it has been useful. Even more so, I hope it has been inspiring and will lead you to take action.

Whether it be by going to visit the dentist, recommending that someone close to you goes, or by downloading a poster and giving it to a place where children play, I hope that this book can help to make a difference.

One other thing I want to do is to raise awareness of the good that is done by Bridge 2 Aid in Africa. By buying this book you have already contributed to the good work they do.

I thank you for that and for reading my book.

About the Author

Alif lives in Leicester with his wife and his beloved daughter Anniyah.

Alif has been a dentist for 10 years and is frequently referred new patients who have been seeing another dentist.

"I'm frequently surprised by how poorly people understand their own mouths and what could happen inside them. I genuinely think that dentists have a responsibility to educate patients and I invest lots of time explaining treatments and treatment options to patients so that they have a better understanding of what's happening. I appreciate that this can be very difficult and time-consuming and often we as dentists are very comfortable talking in 'jargon' so it can be very difficult for patients to understand and comprehend what is going on."

Alif studied at the University of Birmingham School of dentistry and qualified in 2004. Since then he's been working in practice refining his skills and improving his knowledge. He has attended hundreds of courses on a wide variety of topics including provision of different clinical dental treatments like orthodontics, cosmetic dentistry and dental implants, treatments complimentary to dentistry like dermal fillers and Botox and numerous courses that help him communicate more effectively and hence deliver dentistry in a more effective way.

"I feel it is these courses that have enhanced my dentistry more than any others. I think if patients can understand what we're doing and why we are doing it they are much happier and are far more willing to accept treatments that will benefit them more in the long term. Happy patients means a happy dentist."

"People have asked me 'Why did you call your book the smiling dentist when it is for patients and not for dentists?' I explained that I smile most when my patients are happy, especially if they tell me, and even more so if they bring me a present!!'"

Alif's parents are from Tanzania and he's managed to visit there a few times now.

"I'm always sad to see the poverty that some of the world's poorest people have to live in and I think our natural reaction as a human being is to help or at least to want to help. That is why I am so happy to be in the privileged position to be able to donate all of the proceeds of this book to a wonderful charity called Bridge to aid which helps to give some of the poorest people in the world access to dental treatment. Some of whom have been suffering for months before they are able to see somebody to help them with their pain."

I sincerely hope that you enjoyed reading this book and I hope that it helps you. The more people this book helps, whether it be here or in Tanzania, the bigger my smile will be!

Made in the USA
Charleston, SC
31 July 2016